Don't Call Me A Vegan!

Becoming a Vegan is a Personal Choice, however…

**At Age 62 and with What I
Have Learned About the
*Science of Nutrition…***

**I Had No Choice But to Try
Plant-Based Nutrition
And It Works!**

Copyright ©

Contents

Preface

Woody Allen famously said:

"I don't mind dying, I just don't want to be there when it happens."

But the sad truth is, a growing majority of Americans, and those who have adopted our foods and lifestyle, spend the last 10 years of their lives dealing with health issues that are often painful, unpleasant, life-threatening, costly and simply time-wasting of what little time they have left, thereby robbing them of precious moments and quality of life.

Everywhere I go, I seem to see more and more people who can barely walk! They have walkers and canes and wheelchairs, or they waddle, and many seem to struggle and be in pain. I don't remember seeing many people like this when I was younger. None of my grandparents had a cane or a walker.

They must make many visits to medical professionals who walk them along a tightrope of multiple medications that need to be adjusted and balanced and augmented and paid for somehow. And they also must occasionally go into treatment centers, *sometimes in a big hurry*, for medical procedures.

With several health issues myself, I was certainly headed for this kind of future. I was 40 years of age and I was over-weight, such that I was in the "obese" range of the body mass index(BMI); I was prescribed four medications(none of which I took for very long), as I had high blood pressure, high cholesterol, high triglycerides, and a high level of uric acid.

And to make life even less enjoyable, I had the propensity to sweat even after mild exertion. So I started to look for alternative and hopefully better solutions than the phar-maceuticals for which I had been given prescriptions by the physician.

So as I began to look around for alternatives, I ended up trying a number of different things. Mostly being what-ever the latest things (fads) I heard about. Some worked, some didn't, one in particular made things worse.

However with some trial and error and successes, over the next 20 plus years, thankfully, I saw some very good im-provements in my health.

So by the time I was almost age 60, I had managed to get my weight down a total of 40 pounds and to regain some of my youthful vitality. With this vitality, I found an ac-tivity I enjoyed very much: bicycling. So as examples of my vitality, I could and did ride some "Centuries" where I rode my bicycle over 100 miles in a day. And I did it with-out really sweating or getting winded.

I did a multi-day ride across most of the state of Missouri and then three times I did the week long 475 mile ride across the state of Iowa, and three times I did two week fully self supported 500 mile rides across and around Europe. So all in all, I was fairly strong and feeling pretty good and had reasonably good numbers coming back as the results from blood tests.

Compared to most men living in Western civilizations my age I was doing pretty darn good!. But unfortunately, I was still susceptible to some of the effects of some of the medical conditions,

So because I still wasn't satisfied with the progress I had made with my health, I decided to really look into, examine, and learn about the science of what I was consuming and how it affects my body and the way I feel.

So in a nutshell, this book is about what I have found over the last two years of digging into and studying the science. And also, what I have personally experienced by applying this information in the way of "Plant Based Nutrition". Which is what I have been consuming and continue to enjoy to this day.

And I am excited to tell you it has been an amazing transition! I have made a transition from "Pretty Good" to "Remarkably Great"!

I finally was requiring myself to seek out and acquire fact-based evidence rather than just following the latest popular fad. I was feeding myself and my million million cells with credible science based nutrition.

After implementing this decision into practice, now two years later, my weight is down another 25 pounds, my previously unattractive "belly" and "manboobs" are quite a bit smaller, my health issues have either significantly improved or gone away, and I feel amazingly light and energetic.

And I like what I see in the mirror! The inflammation that showed up as puffiness in my face has gone away and people keep telling me how good I look! What a great feeling that is!

It is really hard to describe how good I feel each morning when I wake up. I have an abundance of energy, and feel fantastic! And it gives me even more energy to share this and so I want you to feel this way too!

Looking back over the last two years, what I have done really wasn't that hard once I made the decision to do it. And to be completely honest, I never really felt deprived, hungry or unsatisfied, or restricted like I was trying to live with only limited choices.

On the contrary, I kept feeling more and more satisfied about the way I looked and the way I felt, and I kept finding more and more exciting and yummy foods to eat, so I was motivated to keep doing the things I was doing, and learning, and progressing forward. I eat some really good things! Invite me over, I would love to come and cook for you!

However, in talking with many people, usually because they are interested in asking me how I lost so much weight and look so much better, over the last two years, I think I have a pretty good grasp about what most people think about nutrition, and how they react to something that seems different to them.

It's no wonder—there is so much conflicting information out there—particularly if you just listen to what makes the headlines, the news or the commercials. And of course we all fear the unknown at times.

In general people seem confused. For instance, one person was talking about how water fasting for 12 to 15 days sounded so good to help the body to heal naturally. But later in the conversation she talked about all the supplements and protein powders she was using, which from what I have learned may be overloading her body with processed, isolated substances.

And please, I highly encourage you to dig into this stuff for yourself, it is way too important for your health, vitality and longevity to take this information lightly. And please don't just trust someone like me who took the time to write a book because it "sounds reasonable".

Dig for yourself into the facts and to do that you can use this book as a guide. It's designed to give you quick pathways to valuable information presented by credible people who back it up with real science.

To get you to the heart of the issues as efficiently as possible, I have chosen links to mostly quick videos on subjects by people I have found to be credible presenters of science. And those videos give links to the actual scientific articles that I encourage readers to dive down into themselves.

Best wishes and good luck with your health, vitality and longevity!

"You will either step forward into growth, or you will step backward into safety." - Abraham Maslow
"Twenty years from now you will be more disappointed by the things you didn't do than by the ones you did do. So throw off the bowlines. Sail away from the safe harbor." - Mark Twain

"The best day of your life is the one on which you decide your life is your own, no apologies or excuses. No one to lean on, rely on, or blame. The gift is yours, it is an amazing journey, and you alone
are responsible for the quality of it. This is the day your life really begins." - Allison Atkinson

"You cannot become who you want to be by remaining who you are." - Max Depree

"Nobody ever wrote down a plan to be broke, fat, lazy, or stupid. Those things are what happens when you don't have a plan." - Larry Winget

Introduction

In 1985, while I was in graduate school, I had the wonderful opportunity for a paid internship at the 3M Company at its headquarters in St. Paul, Minn.

For six months, during mosquito season, I was a Strategic Planning intern working with the top executive team that oversaw the Electronics & Information Technology Sector, which at the time accounted for about one-fourth of the operating units and top line for the corporation.

Working under the direction of this team really helped me to learn how to view situations from a higher vantage point -- from a level not mired down in day-to-day requirements and processes.

To help me build upon my ability to see things from a 20- or 30-thousand foot strategic level the team members suggested I read books and articles on warfare strategists Sun Tzu and Napoleon, among others.

They had me read some of the latest business books at the time and write executive summaries for time-challenged sector level and operating unit executive teams.

I learned how the 3M model of innovation and business development works and how it has carried them success-fully through the years. It's an especially impressive accomplishment when you consider that 3M has fared much better than Kodak and Xerox, some of its blue chip rivals back in 1985.

3M allowed scientists and engineers to have 20 percent of their time to be "unassigned." They could freely pursue any innovations that came into their heads, or talk to other engineers or scientists to see what they were doing, possibly not even in the same business sector.

This approach, for instance, is what gave the scientist who invented Post-It notes the free time to play around with adhesive coatings on papers to create page markers for his hymnal when he sang in the church choir.

Then, to pull these innovations out of the labs and the heads of the researchers, the business unit managers were challenged and even required to make sure at least 25 percent of their revenues were generated from products that did not exist five years earlier. These company goals kept a pool full of innovative ideas and offered strong incentives to get them to market.

In 2017 it was reported that 34% of 3M revenue was from products not existing 5 years before. This is a company that makes 50,000 different products so the quantity of new products created continuously is quite impressive.

At 3M, I learned that even when up viewing the landscape

or battlefield at a strategic level the best decisions require facts from down on the ground based upon real science and engineering. Those facts can be about the marketplace or about the technology being applied, but there are techniques to observe and gather information, and proven scientific methods in almost every field that can be applied to data to try and get to the facts, the realities of the situation.

Eye-opening experiences
Well one day, about 2 years ago, I had a moment of clarity about my health. Drawing on those lessons from 3M, I realized that the decisions I was making about my nutrition were not being made up at the strategic level, and I certainly had not been rigorous in making sure I had collected and mentally processed the best scientifically proven facts I could find before making my decisions and choices.

I was like a blind man with an elephant trying to figure out what kind of animal it was. I would go around touching different parts of the elephant, and each touch would give me a different impression of what I was feeling. Depending on which part of the animal I was touching I thought I was dealing with different animals.

So instead of having a complete view allowing me to make well considered choices, I got enough partial information to then "wing it" and try different popular ideas or "fads", so to speak, about my health. Dealing more with different component parts of nutrition and my health instead of the whole big picture.

What I needed to do was to rise up and open my eyes to really see what I was dealing with, and then to try to collect the best science about my health so I could deal with it in a way for the best long-term outcomes.

For the last two years I have been obsessed with finding the best peer-reviewed scientific information available about what impact nutrition has on an individual human body, its processes and cells, on how nutrition affects different populations, on how the various marketplace forces affect the foods we eat, and if possible, how that information can be organized to create a strategic view.

I'm now ready to share this scientifically based view. I know it has helped me to feel better, and have better blood test numbers, and to take my health up another level or two or three!

I will assume in your lives, you are essentially very busy "executives" with hundreds of things to be done or on your mind, and many of you may have not had any "business reason" yet to seek out answers about health issues or feel the need to seek and pull innovative ideas out of the scientifically valid pool created by the researchers.

But I'm sure that some of you have had reasons. I call these "taps of the health hammer" on the head. Hopefully, they have been a gentle wake-up taps, because I know people who have been walloped. I myself had at least four taps on the head: one of them very painful, one of them unpleasant and concerning, and all of them embarrassing and deflating to my ego.

All of them just made life less enjoyable.

With the percentages that are documented on the prevalence of each of these four health issues in our society today, the odds are that almost everyone reading this book
has at least one of these issues, or most likely, has a loved
one with one or more of these issues.

**Someone you know, love, or care for, or your own health,
your longevity, or your ability to avoid pain, may depend
upon having this information, perspective and strategic
viewpoint and the opportunity for innovation with nutrition.**

Personally I grew up eating like a glutenous caveman. I
did successfully reproduce in my 30s, so my "propagating
the species" job was done and I passed on my genes to the
next generation of thankfully born healthy children. But
my omnivore/processed foods ways started to cause sick-
ness in my 40s.

So I started a journey looking for answers which has now
led me to what is essentially the "Science of Longevity".
And in learning this science I have discovered there is a
low risk/high reward wager that can be made with health.
Making this wager, essentially with pennies in direct costs,
has led me to feeling good every day, with my body being
able to serve as my host for as long as possible without
malfunctioning.

It is incredibly low cost, high profit, and has virtually no
side effects. If this was a patentable pharmaceutical I think
the manufacturer would have the highest market cap on
the NYSE.

Executive Summary

- Like the general population, the number one cause of death of cardiologists in America is heart disease. So heart doctors are no different than the rest of us in that regard. These professionals are trained to apply medical procedures and pharmaceuticals yet do not seem to have any special answers for their and our number one cause of death.

  So the question I ask you to put into your mind is: "If the number one cause of death of airline pilots was plane crashes, how would you feel about getting on a commercial flight?" (If you're a fearful flier, rest assured—their main cause of death, like the rest of us, is heart disease. But you get the point.)

- The surface area of our skin is quite large and many people take great care of how it interacts with their environment. The surface area of our digestive tract is much larger, about the size of a tennis court. Most people take great care to make sure their skin does not become inflamed by overexposure to the sun.

But there is a large amount of scientific evidence that the typical American diet is very inflammatory. But because it is hidden, unlike our skin, we do not see the "sunburns" we are causing with each of our typical American meals and snacks.

– The surface area of our entire cardiovascular system is also huge, at about the size of seven tennis courts and is lined by cells that are only one cell thick. That one cell thin layer is called the Endothelium and once again this important layer is subject to inflammation and other types of direct damage done by the types of foods that are typically consumed in Western cultures.

Many common fatal, debilitating and painful diseases have their roots in this damage to the lining and walls of our cardiovascular systems.

– Many of what are now the most common causes of diseases and premature death in the United States were rare before the industrialization of our food supply.

The epidemic rates of coronary heart disease, brain diseases, digestive cancers, infections, type 2 diabetes, high blood pressure, liver disease, blood cancers, kidney disease, breast cancer, suicidal depression, prostate cancer, autoimmune diseases, and even lung diseases have risen as our society consumes industrially produced food.

Population studies from around the world have confirmed similar experiences as others have adopted our processed foods diet and they also confirm that societies where they have not adopted our ways still have low incidences of these "lifestyle diseases."

– As should be expected, the food industries make great efforts to promote their businesses and protect their investments. Also they often receive the help of federal and state governments which have departments with mandates to help the country's important industries be successful and grow.

There are a lot of similarities with the tobacco industry on how the emerging scientific facts and industry interests are in conflict, and the food industry seems to be using many of the same defensive strategies and tactics to protect their business and investments.

– The modern business model is very much about creating products that are scalable. A venture capitalist, or a business unit manager at 3M, is going to analyze the market size, how many units can be produced, what percentage of the market can be captured, etc.

So you have to have a "product", something that can be reduced down into a "unit" that can be "manufactured" and reproduced in mass quantities that are further protected with patents, copyrights, branding, secret formulas, and so on.

Therefore the food, pharmaceutical, supplement, medical procedure, and even the "health advice" industries are naturally interested in massive scale and growth by making and selling more units.

- Medical care is not "Health Care", rather it is "Sick Care". The units being sold by this industry very rarely "cure" anyone taking them. True "health" is not restored.

  They may keep you alive, they may get you past the episode or attack that caused you to seek help, but they do not cure. Ask your cardiologist how long you have to take any of the various statin drugs and he (or she) will likely tell you to take them for the rest of your life.

- Human cells regenerate on average about every 100 days. This is hard for some people to grasp because they don't see any changes when they look at themselves over the short term. But they really do.

  There is an abundance of peer-reviewed scientific evidence to show which substances assist our cells in successful regeneration and which ones cause our cells to mutate, not reproduce at all, just die off, or to possibly cause the growth of mutated cells into things like deadly cancers.

- The bacteria in our gut feeds on what we consume. What it is fed and the substances its various "colonies" produce inside of us are proving to be very important in how our bodies work and age and how we feel physically and mentally.

  One of the more intriguing recent discoveries has to do

with the role of the gut microbiome, the trillions of microbes that reside in the GI (gastrointestinal) tract, and how they influence our health by helping digest food, producing vitamins and other chemicals, and hopefully providing protection against disease-causing micro-organisms.

What we consume feeds the various colonies of "bugs" in our digestive tract and science is learning which foods feed and grow colonies producing beneficial substances and which produce harmful substances.

– Blood flow is so very important to most of our systems. Of course it is obvious that any interruption of blood flow to the heart, brain, or penis can cause dramatic unpleasant effects. But more fundamentally the blood provides the primary transport for the chemicals that supply our cells in their efforts to regenerate successfully.

These chemicals make up the environment in which the cells exist and that environment influences how our genes express themselves, either positively or negatively. Even our joints seem to be failing sooner because of poor blood delivery.

– How the body deals with and eliminates toxins is very important. Without effective elimination, toxins can recycle through our systems and build up. The liver does much of the heavy lifting in detoxifying by filtering waste out of our blood.

It produces bile acids and salts that contain these filtered out toxins, sending them over to the gallbladder, a little muscular sac, which then pumps them into our small intestine just below the stomach. It's all part of our digestive process.

Some of these toxins are then reabsorbed by the small or large intestine. But how much is reabsorbed versus how much is eliminated via our stools has to do with the bile binding ability of the fiber we eat.

So unfortunately most Americans are recycling more toxins through their bodies than is desirable because 96% of us do not consume even the minimum recommended amount of fiber. This recycling of toxins builds up the gunk that forms painful gallstones and burns out the gallbladder which is why so many of them are being removed these days.

– Epidemic of "Diabesity". Fifty per cent of Americans are either diabetic or pre-diabetic. For example, 70% of people who apply for military service are rejected for weight related issues.

Our bodies were not engineered by the evolutionary process to properly handle the excess substances that race into our systems when we consume processed foods. Evolution engineered us to be able to survive long enough to reproduce, that is the basic process of natural selection.

One of those survival tools is to store resources any

time we get more than the body needs to currently function, just in case of famine. So with the typical American processed nutrition, the body is constantly trying to store the excess waves that hit it with every meal and snack.

The body was engineered to do the processing itself, which slows the way the substances go into our systems. Cavemen did not have blenders or juicers. They chewed.

- Humans have the "ability" to be Omnivores, eating like cavemen did for survival. That contributed to what got our species here today through some pretty rough conditions. But to keep the species going through the eras and eons, humans and their predecessors, the great apes, only had to live long enough to reproduce.

So the "science" presented to justify eating Omnivore or Paleo is the science of cavepeople survival, to eat whatever they could find or kill, but whose life expectancy was about 35 years or so. But if longevity and long term vitality are your goal then science points in a different direction.

- So in some ways, it is like 1964 all over again. Then it was tobacco, now it is nutrition. Cigarette smoking peaked in 1964, and has been declining ever since. The watershed event was when the Surgeon General of the United States brought to light the scientific research on the negative health effects of smoking.

Some of this research on tobacco had been around since the 1930s, but it took until 1964 for the governmental authorities to make an authoritative statement about it.

There is now also decades of scientific research out there about how the typical American diet is causing numerous "lifestyle diseases" and there is a core group of dedicated scientists and health care professionals trying to bring it to the public consciousness, currently without the help of the authorities. But scientific facts don't go away, and ignoring them can be perilous to your health.

– Chronic inflammation and immune system responses from our nutritional choices seem to be the root cause of premature aging as well as so very many symptoms that are huge market opportunities for the pharmaceutical, medical, supplements, over the counter treatment, and "dietary solution" industries.

Digestive issue symptoms are a very good example. So many providers of solutions from all the above industries are lined up waiting to sell "solutions" which help relieve symptoms. None of them really "cure" the "diseases".

Occasionally a dietary choice is identified and modified providing some relief, such as with gluten intolerance or Celiac disease. The real underlying cause is still not resolved, it just lessens the symptoms.

In my opinion, taking a 20-to30-thousand foot strategic view, it's still the preponderance of processed inflammatory foods in our typical diets that are the root cause of such a dramatic rise in diseases, allergies and intolerances such as gluten, heart disease, diabetes, high blood pressure, etc.

– Even if a person consumes the absolute best "high quality protein" from animals that is supposedly free of antibiotics, toxins and contaminants, or whatever, there is "baggage" brought into the body with the protein.

Even the type of iron found in animal flesh, Heme Iron, races into the human body in an unregulated manner potentially causing harm. And then when undigested particles of the protein progress to the large intestine, they are digested by the anerobic bacteria producing toxic hydrogen sulfide gas which is linked to bowel diseases and a substance called TMAO which is linked to cardiovascular diseases.

There is an "endgame" to be considered. There is a very worthwhile goal in my humble opinion. And one that I feel very strongly that I have experienced.

That being the changeover of the trillions of cells in the gut microbiome from being dominated by colonies that are producing chemicals that are inflammatory, toxic and disease promoting, to colonies that provide beneficial chemicals that are nurturing and provide a good environment for our bodies cell regeneration processes.

Based on some factors I have noticed about myself, I have made this transition ... and it feels great! So in this book I will show you some ways to "move the ball down the field" to better health, and show you how I think I have made it to the "end zone" which is always a happy and exciting place to be and to celebrate!

– There is proven and peer reviewed scientific evidence and clinical experience documented to show that there are nutritional choices that can arrest the development and growth of mutations and to even reverse some of the effects.

But so far none of this knowledge has been distilled down into a unit such as a pill or a procedure that can be produced, packaged, marketed and sold in a scalable way to produce the results that will fit into the modern business model.

But to re-emphasize this important point: these diseases do not have to happen and they are clinically being shown they can be stopped and reversed.

– There is a significant potential opportunity in working with the expense side of the current business model when it comes to out of control healthcare costs, which are putting a huge burden on society and individual enterprises.

There is a growing body of both scientific and clinical

experience that some costly afflictions can be rapidly
reversed, with notable progress even in a few weeks.
Given the proper attention, this significant improvement and savings could gain the attention of enterprises looking for relatively quick quarter to quarter improvement in cost control.

I Had so Many Questions

Why was I taking fish oil pills? For the Omega 3s? But why really? And were there only positives to taking them, or were there negatives?

Are "free range" or "cage free" eggs better? Why?

Was it worth it to spend extra money to buy wild caught Salmon?

What does "grass fed" mean and does it make any difference?

Is it worth spending extra on free range antibiotic free chicken?

Why was everyone talking about where they were getting their high quality protein? Are some proteins better than others? What does protein really do for us anyway? I've never heard of anyone coming home from the doctor having been told they were protein deficient (unless they just weren't eating enough like an elderly or anorexic person), yet people seem to be concerned about it.

My blood tests over the last few years indicated I was at

the low end of the range for vitamin D. Is that because I don't spend enough time in the sun? But every carton of milk I have ever seen or consumed since I was in kindergarten has said it contained vitamin D so how could I be deficient?

Why were many of our restaurant customers avoiding gluten?

What did cave people really eat and were they healthy? How long did they live?

I know that I didn't have any "scientific" basis for trying the Keto diet 22 years ago when it was called the Atkins Diet?

I had heard about "Blue Zones" where people live long and healthy. They all seemed to be near the ocean, so I assumed it must be because of eating fish. So I took more fish oil and ate a lot of salmon. But I made assumptions and did not take the time to actually read the books. I didn't find out why.

I was making so many decisions about what I bought and consumed but when I really and truthfully tried to answer the question: "How did I know?"   I had to admit I really didn't know for sure.

Why did I blindly take meds prescribed by doctors without taking the time to research, read and understand the potential side effects?

I seemed to be assuming a lot. And I'm sure I wasn't alone.

Most Likely I Have Been Where You Are Now

I was the kid eating hamburgers, hot dogs, pizza, mac and cheese, fries, drinking sugary Kool Aid® and Hi-C® and Coke® and Pepsi.®

As a teenager, I was drinking soda and beer, eating massive amounts of junk food, and gained 50 pounds my freshman year in college. Yes 50 not 15.

I was the young man now with a degree working and travelling and continuing to consume food like a drunk teenager at college, but with more money.

Then in my 20s I ended up in the hospital with severe abdominal pains. With lots of tests and no explanation, I was admitted for 5 days. Still with no explanation, I finally got relief after a barium enema must have flushed out whatever it was that was causing the pain.

And it goes on and on. I had the beginnings of many unpleasant diseases that are all now very common in our society today.

You can see that I know how rough, uncomfortable and downright painful the journey can be, but I also know there is a path that really isn't that difficult that can get me (health wise) to a safer better place. And that path is low risk, low cost, and with almost no danger from side effects.

So I was where you may be, but I have been working to get up ahead, hacking my way through the thicket of pseudo-science, looking for answers based on science and now sending word back to the group as to what I have experienced and seen, what I have learned about the opposing forces, and which path will offer the least resistance with the least amount of damage for anyone who might want to follow.

Doing More Research on What Kind of Car to Buy

I realized I was doing more research on where to go on vacation, or what kind of car to buy, or even where to go for dinner than on what choices I was making about what to put into my body; the one and only body I have in this one life with which I have been blessed.

Then a moment of clarity occurred when I finally realized that I was swimming, floating and possibly drowning in a constant flow of "messages" about nutrition and health and I was grabbing on to some of it that seemed to make sense.

What made sense to me was based upon and through the filters of what I had experienced and been taught over the course of my life by people who probably didn't really know why they consumed what they did either.

When I really stopped and tried to view it all from an objective perspective, I realized I was making choices with no proven science behind the information I was using to make those many food decisions and choices. Our bodies are biochemical and mechanical machines so I figured there must be some proven science out there.

It seemed like every other week there was a new headline with new information that I was using to factor into my decision making about my choices. Sound familiar?

I had suffered through some unpleasant and/or painful "wake up calls" concerning my health already in my life. Each time I went looking on the world wide web for "causes."

Sources such as the MayoClinic.org or WebMD.com always mentioned food and drinks as possibly contributing to my unhappiness from these unpleasant conditions. So it just seemed logical that I look more into the things I could control. I couldn't change my genetics, but I could try to find the best information about what I consumed.

I can't change the genetics that gave me red hair and skin that sunburns quickly. But I can control how much of the sun's rays come into contact with my skin causing potentially painful and long term damage.

So someone who rationalizes that they are destined to certain health problems because of genetics should step back and look at the logic of that rationalization and the available science.

Getting Good Information When Making Choices

I try to make good choices, but I'm human and give in to temptation like everyone does when there are "impulse items" available to grab on either side of the aisle and on the "end caps" as I approach the "cash register at the grocery store of life".

Napoleon Hill, one of the most widely published "self-help" authors of all time, has a list of "Ten Rules of Self Discipline", and number six on the list is: "Learn to ask questions and listen to the answers" especially: "How do you know?" In a recorded talk he emphasized asking the question: "How do you know?" anytime someone is trying to pass something off to you as true.

When I started to apply this question to things I was doing or thought, it made me realize that **I did not really "know" ... I had not been rigorous in the pursuit of evidence to prove why I should believe and/or do something.**

So I suggest when you hear or read the latest headline where a magazine, newspaper, article on the internet, or a news reader references "the latest study" or "a new book out" or whatever, that you question whether your source has taken the time to drill into this latest thing to see if it is credible and to see "how did they know". Or did they just pass on some concept they hope will catch your eye and get you to buy a copy or click on their web page.

The Last "Diet Concept" I Considered
Before Seeking the Science

So many fads and theories and things that sounded reasonable had come and gone as I moved along my journey ... but for this last one my wife had bought the books Grain Brain and Wheat Belly and read them and bought into them because people at the health club were talking about them and how much those people said they had been helped.

So I picked up the books, scanned and read parts of them to get the key points, and thought they made some sense, so I started to cut back on wheat and gluten etc.—sound familiar?

But did I really look into the sources cited by the authors or try to see if their conclusions had any credible science backing them up? No, I didn't. I would be willing to bet most people didn't.

But I was willing to change my nutrition, like many people, based on what seemed to sound right. But that's quite different from applying the question: "How do you know?"

I have to admit that the 2 books about grain, wheat and gluten did help us, especially my wife who, like many women, had been suffering from varying amounts of intestinal discomfort over the years. And cutting down on the products that contain gluten, and by cutting down on processed foods in general, moved us along the path to better health.

But was it the gluten? What about the other "stuff" that may be in "baked goods"? Such as: Bromated flour, genetically modified substances, fields of wheat sprayed with pesticides, and on and on.

Or were our digestive systems just so inflamed from the eggs and cheese and meat and processed foods so that products with gluten caused a noticeable unpleasant irritation? What was the actual source of the problem? The body is an amazingly complex interrelated set of systems, and as I am learning, there are so many other factors to consider.

But I had other health issues going on so I didn't stop there. And because I kept digging for peer-reviewed scientifically proven evidence and learning, I now realize there is so much more going on with our bodies.

Even though there was anecdotal progress made by reducing the products that contained gluten, and especially some relief in my wife's symptoms, I concluded that trying someone's theory that focused on one nutritional input, there could be even better progress and relief by getting to the possible root causes rather than looking at just one single symptom, and one single food element.

Paleo is another theory that can have good benefits for some people by getting them off of processed foods. But I have learned by now there is "baggage" that comes along with some of the benefits.

Information is Out There
and is Accessible

In my search, I have learned to dig into the sources and the credentials of the authors of the studies. Even if they are peer-reviewed, there can be conflicts of interest.

https://nutritionfacts.org/video/disclosing-conflicts-interest-medical-research/
https://nutritionfacts.org/video/eliminating-conflicts-of-interest-in-medical-research/

Even well-known "charitable organizations" seem to have conflicts of interest because they are accepting corporate sponsorship money.
https://www.laprogressive.com/cancer-charities/

You may have noticed by this point that I am a huge fan of the internet, and the access it gives us to information. Just as an example, I have been jumping onto MIT's Open Courseware for years at https://ocw.mit.edu/index.htm for fun and amusement whenever my brain thought of a subject I was curious about.

Like electrical engineering, which I have been interested in since I was a kid, and started to pursue in college, but then took a different path. Nonetheless, I am still a science geek at heart.

It Started When We Had a Badly Disturbing Evening Watching Netflix

We had heard through family chit-chat that one of our daughters was trying "Veganism" after watching a couple of documentaries on Netflix, and that she was having some success with her weight and her complexion.

So on Sunday August 6, 2017, we watched two documentaries and they made sense, although they also grossed us out about the way animal products are raised.

We decided mainly because of the "yuck" factor to try it. The thought of continuing to eat food that is basically raised in its own filth and is often times sick and suffering just was no longer appetizing to us.

I immediately texted our nephew in Portland, Oregon. He had been a Vegan at times. I asked him for some tips on going "Vegan."

Based on his advice, I tried some things, and I felt better, and some things quickly changed, and I felt different, but did I know why? No, not at all, I had not yet applied the question: "How do you know?" At that point it was just the next popular thing we had heard about to try, like I had done with Atkins, vegetarianism, fish oil pills, seaweed and kelp, gluten, etc.

But even after just a few weeks I was feeling surprisingly better and some pounds had melted off without counting calories or peeing on test strips. I was eating delicious foods in quantities that kept me satisfied, and so I had an "uh huh" and a "hmmmm" moment or two.

So I decided I wasn't going to let this just be the next fad that came along that seemed to make sense. I have a computer with access to a wealth of information on the internet, I know how to do research, so I became obsessed, and still am, with finding supportable scientific information.

I never really liked biology or chemistry in high school. Maybe it was the instructors I had, or maybe it just wasn't the way my brain works. I was a physics guy, enjoyed electricity and stuff like that … but what I have been learning now is basically biochemistry, biomechanics, nutritional anthropology, evolution, genetics, and populations.

It required some perseverance and diving and digging, but I have found that real supportable information does exist. However, I have also discovered there is also a lot of "sounds reasonable" yet not scientifically supported "information" out there too. And salespeople are pushing information for profit.

So in my humble opinion, there is an "oily film" of misinformation up on the surface of the sea of knowledge about human nutrition science.

This is what I have learned, and what I have experienced, what I have tried myself, in as concise and informative a way as I can so (hopefully) you will at least humor me enough to spend a little time to read and contemplate this information for yourself. And maybe even be inspired enough to try science based nutrition.

As I have said, there aren't any potential dangerous side effects like there are with taking some medications or starving the body with some of the fad diets. Just upsides and feeling better.

But a key point is I had made some improvements and I was being and feeling pretty healthy for quite a few years before I started to transition to nutrition based upon the science of longevity.

I was eating well (lots of seafood, almost no red meat, chicken once in a while. I was getting plenty of high quality protein), **getting some exercise** (I was able to ride "Centuries" - 100 miles or more in a day on a bicycle), **my numbers were good** (my blood pressure was rock solid, cholesterol was ok, my checkups were very good for being an almost 60 year old American male) and at my **age to not be taking any medications** was already excellent.

Sure I had pizza once in a while, but **I was basically doing the Mediterranean diet and more and more was buying organic, free range, wild caught etc. ...** and I really thought

I felt pretty good … but, once I tried this new path, things changed about my body and the way it functioned and the way I felt, and so **things began to reveal themselves to me.**

Mostly what has been revealed is about how much better I could feel (it is truly hard to describe how much better and lighter and cleaner I feel) and how much better my numbers could be, and how much of a better chance I am giving myself to live a long pain free life.

One of the first things I noticed was that first trip down the stairs in the morning where, even when I thought I was feeling and doing so good, I would have some stiffness in my feet and knees. I had previously gotten used to it thinking it was normal and inevitable…..I thought it was just aging, but it went away after a few weeks!

Biochemistry
As you probably are aware, you can find just about everything on YouTube, from fixing your dryer, to how to meditate. So of course I appreciate you are all very busy people, which is why I have links to videos instead of links to the actual scientific sources which most people will not link to and read.

But the videos I am choosing mostly all have direct links in them to the published scientific papers cited in the videos. So if you have the time and inclination you can drill down too.

Admittedly this is not a book of original research but instead a framework of thought that hopefully provides an understanding by directing the reader to information. The open minded may form a different way of looking at the subject of nutrition. So thank you to all the people who have created the research and the content that I am high-lighting in order to give the reader a new perspective.

I have spent a lot of time over the last two years clicking on the sources cited by the Vloggers to create my own Master-class or program in the science of how nutrition affects our bodies, and most importantly, how it provides the chemical and biological requirements that are optimal for our amazing bodies.

Nutrition allows our systems to maintain and repair them-selves, and to function in a way to avoid the most suffering from diseases, some of which I have already personally ex-perienced and do not want to experience anymore.

But the subject at hand when one really gets down to it is Biochemistry. And whether you go to the paper based li-brary or use the internet, there is peer-reviewed literature that presents research work done using scientific methods.

My Background

A nd so as a 17 year old I didn't make it very far in the Engineering Physics program at the University of Illinois at Urbana Champaign.

I then side-shifted into and through the Accounting program at Illinois State and the MBA program at the University of Illinois at Chicago, and therefore don't have any real degreed cred in biochemistry, but I can still read and use my eyes and brain to figure out which nutrition "science" out there is credible or just someone's hypothesis and not really "put to the test" of serious rigorous scientific methods and therefore presented in credible peer reviewed journals.

But as a note, I did get a full ride for graduate school as a research assistant and also did the aforementioned six month strategic planning internship at 3M where I did some pretty interesting industry research that was supplied to the executive teams on current hot business and technology topics.

I was researching the emerging science of flat panel displays when the projection TVs were the show off items in the man caves. So I have some experience digging and learning.

And the education I received in learning how to pass the CPA exam taught me how to "audit" both quantitatively and qualitatively, and to use statistical sampling to project the results of sampling to larger populations. And how to critically read and understand statistics.

And as a Management Consultant with one of the world's largest consulting firms, I learned "process consulting" where almost everything can be broken down into processes and then viewed objectively.

And how to look at things and situations strategically from different viewpoints and levels of observation. And, how to really separate my own preconceived ideas from the situation at hand and to just lay the cards out on the table so to speak to really try and see what is going on.

So please give my writing a chance, (because I have spent 2 years now trying to drill past the industry funded "science" and the books written based on unproven hypothesis), and read this book that I've taken the time to write, and think about it, and maybe try some things......but at least please for your own potential benefit, try to read it and think about it.

And even if you don't read this book for yourself, please at least read it in consideration of someone else you may be caring for and feeding. This is the best science I can find so far about providing nutrition to humans.

I am a father and a grandfather, and a person who doesn't like pain and suffering, trying to find and get my head around the best most factual science there is about nutrition and how it affects human bodies.

I am about personal choice. But I am about getting the facts. And I think I have been getting to them.

Science aside, this is about life and vitality and especially about not suffering during the last ten years of life ... and so the best terms I have come across that describe the path I am on are Nutrivore or Nutritarian, which to me is about learning the best and latest science about nutrition and then making personal choices and positive changes.

This is vital to your future and quality of life.

To whet your appetite for skepticism about what you think you "know", but has actually been fed to you as a steady diet since childhood, check out this eye-opening video on strategies and tactics used by the Tobacco and Food Industries:
https://www.youtube.com/watch?v=J9vpohU4-zo

Scientific Method

As a refresher, let me review the "scientific method," which has been around since the 17th century, and particularly look at how it relates to ideas about nutrition.

So to start, someone has a question they would like to try to answer, or, they make an observation.

From there they construct a hypothesis and test it with one or more experiments.

Then they analyze the results of the experiments to see if they even worked correctly. If not then they circle back and try to fix what went wrong.

Once they think the experiment worked properly, they analyze the results of the experiments and try to draw conclusions.

Then they try to determine if the results supported or refuted the original hypothesis or maybe just caused more questions to be asked. Maybe the process created more observations or questions that needed to be tested.

So there can be multiple loops back to ask more questions, create more hypotheses, and/or try different experiments or go down different paths.

So things can get complicated, and no one is perfect, which is why serious scientific work is subject to "peer review" to help make sure the scientists in the middle of the process don't miss anything and follow sound logic and procedures.

What "peer review" means

So by the time something is published in a peer reviewed journal of some sort, the scientific methods used have likely been reviewed multiple times by colleagues, by department chairpersons, by department review committees, by board level review committees (no institution wants to be embarrassed by putting out erroneous or misguided research papers), and then when the papers are submitted to the journals then they have their own review procedures where independent peers review and try to "shoot holes" in the science being presented.

So getting research findings published in a well-regarded peer-reviewed scientific journal of any kind is a carefully examined process. And if you happen to know any research scientists personally you will probably come to realize they are very critical people.

They like to disagree, and like to shoot down the ideas of others. At cocktail parties they are usually very interesting to talk to but usually end up getting into an argument.

In short, getting peer reviewed research published is like crawling on your belly through a battlefield with bullets whizzing over your head.

On the other hand, writing a book based on someone's ideas, and making some interesting arguments that catch people's attention and "seem to make sense" and getting it published, has a rigor of its own, but the science itself is a lot less rigorous process. Best seller lists are made up of authors who can sell books, regardless of the science contained within.

The stops along my journey looking for solutions to my physical ailments have included Atkins (keto), Grain Brain (gluten free), Paleo (survival), Vegetarianism, Mediterranean Diet, etc.

But now that I have seen the difference between concepts that have been "put to the test" by the scientific method, and those of "interesting ideas" or "hypothesis" that are not supported by the rigorous testing of the full scientific method, well, I think about all this very differently and skeptically.

I've looked at the science of studying the statistical data on the health experiences of different populations around the world, down to the ever opening up science at the microscopic, cellular, and even sub cellular levels.

But to me, the most interesting research is how all the systems of cells in our bodies interact and work together to play a symphony of processes to make our bodies function. For instance, the chemicals produced by our gut bacteria even seem to influence the functioning of our brains.

Beat the Dealer

In the early 1980s I was trading stock index futures, at my broker's office in the Chicago Mercantile Exchange Building. One of my fellow traders turned out to be a professional gambler, playing mostly poker. Day trading futures was one of the ways he amused himself between sessions at card tables.

I was about to fly to Las Vegas for the weekend, so I asked him for any tips he could give me on gambling.

He suggested a book called "Beat the Dealer" which was written by a math professor about using the science of numbers and probabilities to improve your odds at black-jack. https://en.wikipedia.org/wiki/Edward_O._Thorp

I could have just played blackjack and let the cards fall where they may, and accept my losses or winnings. But I wanted to improve my odds so I learned about the science of probabilities and mathematics. It improved my "odds."

So just like with gambling, I thought, why not learn the science to do what I can do to improve the odds with the one body I have been given?

Regardless of my genetic "cards," I'm trying to use scientific knowledge and objective learning to improve my odds. I hope you'll join me.

The Human Body is an Amazingly Complex Symphony of Processes

Our bodies are amazingly complex systems where over 1000 metabolic processes are taking place ... with millions and billions and trillions of cells all needing to be fed and function and supply and regenerate and interact with each other.

There are trillions of cells in each of our digestive tracts that aren't even part of our bodies. We are their hosts, feeding them. And they in return generate and put things back into us, and help things get out of us.

So think about this: medications, drugs, pills, whatever you call them are usually some isolated molecule or two that can be patented and legally protected so the creator can invest in all the research and the processes to synthesize, bottle, market and distribute in a way that hopefully helps some people and creates a profit for the creator.

To think a single molecule or two can comprehensively help someone to be healthy is just not logical. They are thought to attack the specific problem they were created for and leave everything else alone, but have you seen the lists of potential side effects for most medications? They don't leave everything else alone, there are rippling effects throughout our bodies.

To think that focusing on a single nutritional element such as carbohydrates or protein or cholesterol or fat will provide for long term health and vitality also does not take into consideration the amazingly complex nature of all the various chemical, biological and physical processes in the human body.

The "R" Word

The term for trying to apply something simple like a medication or a modification of a single nutritional element like carbs or gluten is **"reductionism."**

Highly acclaimed Cornell University biochemistry researcher Dr. T. Colin Campbell puts it this way:

> *"The fact that each nutrient passes through such a maze of reaction pathways suggests that each nutrient also is likely to participate in multiple health and disease outcomes. The one nutrient/one disease relationship implied by **reductionism**, although widely popular, is simply incorrect. Every nutrient-like chemical that enters this complex system of reactions creates a rippling effect that may extend far into the pool of metabolism. And with every bite of food we eat, there are tens and probably hundreds of thousands of food chemicals entering this metabolism pool more or less simultaneously."*

So the subject of how our body functions is not simple, but we have been approaching our health and vitality looking for simplified solutions as if it was....even as our collective health issues continue mounting.

History of These Now Common Health Problems

Remember the TV show, Lifestyles of the Rich and Famous? Well the more I do research on the common health issues of today, the more I think there should be a show called: The Lifestyle Diseases of the Rich and Famous.

And while many of us may not be famous, many and possibly most of us now are rich enough monetarily and therefore have enough money to afford to get the diseases that used to only affect royalty and the otherwise wealthy. https://www.ncbi.nlm.nih.gov/pubmed/17245475

Poor rural people in Central Africa, where we all came from about 200,000 years ago, do not have these health problems because they can only afford to eat the traditional foods that are similar to what our ancestors ate 10,000 generations before.

Dr. Greger lists the top 15 ways American's die:

- Coronary Heart Disease
- Lung Diseases

- Brain Diseases
- Digestive Cancers
- Infections
- Type 2 Diabetes
- High Blood Pressure
- Liver Disease
- Blood Cancers
- Kidney Disease
- Breast Cancer
- Suicidal Depression
- Prostate Cancer
- Parkinson's Disease
- Medical Care (not including medical errors and mistakes)

https://nutritionfacts.org/video/uprooting-the-leading-causes-of-death/

It seems from the science that most of these things are self-inflicted.

Yes, they can still happen even if a person does everything perfectly, but the rates at which they are attacking us are increasing due to our lifestyle choices and mostly nutritional choices.

https://my.clevelandclinic.org/health/transcripts/1444_lifestyle-choices-root-causes-of-chronic-diseases

Heard About the "Blue Zones"

In the late 1980s when I worked as a Management Consultant we often studied other industries and even competitors to identify "Best Practices" and then used the information to help our clients become more competitive.

Blue Zones follow a similar principle. People living in Blue Zones live, on average, 12 quality healthy years longer than the rest of us do.

Author, explorer, and world record setting long range cyclist, Dan Buettner in conjunction with the highly regarded National Geographic organization and a couple of well-known universities, set out to identify why some areas in the world have people who live longer and with better health than the rest of us.
https://www.bluezones.com/dan-buettner/

When I first heard about the 5 Blue Zones they identified, I assumed it was because they were in areas where seafood was consumed regularly. I was taking fish oil pills at the time, although I didn't really know anything about the science of why.

But my intuition was very wrong. As it turns out, beans, including fava, black, soy and lentils, are the cornerstone of most centenarian diets in these areas. Meat—mostly pork—is eaten on average only five times per month. Serving sizes are 3-4 oz., about the size of a deck of cards.

In one area, Okinawa, Japan, sweet potatoes were the cornerstone of their diet. Beans and sweet potatoes are starches, really healthy starches. They also have lots of phytonutrients to feed the body's complex metabolic processes, and fiber to help the body rid itself of toxins.

You may be thinking that beans and sweet potatoes would lead to a carbohydrate overload, but you would be wrong. That's how thoroughly you've been indoctrinated by the pseudo-science marketers who want you to take their shakes and pills rather than eat good health-providing natural food.

Complex carbohydrates are packed with fiber, phytonutrients, and other elements that are great for your body—and that simply cannot be reproduced in a laboratory.

The Okinawan whole food sweet potato consumption is much different from the processed sweet potato fries that most Americans eat. Processed foods, especially those combined with processed oils essentially race into our systems in ways that our bodies were not developed by 20 million years of natural selection and development to handle correctly for health.

I highly recommend everyone to go out and read Dan's book about the Blue Zones. Very mind expanding stuff about lifestyles in general and not just food.

The nine lessons or best practices of the Blue Zones are:

1. **Move naturally**. Don't do marathons or pump iron; work around the house, garden, walk, cycle, walk when talking on the phone.
2. **Know your purpose**. Have a reason for waking up in the morning.
3. **Kick back**. Find ways to shed stress, whether it's praying, napping or going to happy hour.
4. **Eat less**. Try to stop eating when you are 80% full.
5. **Eat less meat**. Beans are a cornerstone of most centenarians' diets.
6. **Drink in moderation**. Of all the Blue Zones, only the Seventh-day Adventists in California didn't have one to two glasses a day.
7. **Have faith**. Denomination doesn't seem to matter, but attending faith-based services (4 times a month) does.
8. **Power of love**. Put families first, including committing to a partner and keeping aging parents and grandparents nearby.
9. **Stay social**. Build a social network that supports healthy behaviors.

How to Live to be 100+:
https://www.youtube.com/watch?v=ff40YiMmVkU

Living 10 healthy years longer:
https://www.youtube.com/watch?v=KarE7tsVAW4

Journey into the Blue Zone:

https://www.youtube.com/watch?v=Zv0_y1FVW0c

Longevity Secrets of the Loma Linda Blue Zone:
https://www.youtube.com/watch?v=zhJl-T_AB6A

Healthy Aging in Loma Linda
https://www.youtube.com/watch?v=wlIPAvZospo

So for those of you still Looking for a "Silver Bullet" …
… Blue Zones and Wine:
https://www.bluezones.com/2018/02/drinking-glass-wine-taking-walk-may-be-key-to-longevity/

Looking for Studies on the
Health of Populations

While the Blue Zone project sought to find the longest living healthiest people, there are numerous studies that look at populations to try and identify how various factors influence health outcomes.

Some of these studies are quite large and have been going on for many years. And as I kept looking for more and more of these types of studies and digging deeper into the references and the analysis of them I kept realizing they were all leading me to pretty much the same place.

The Adventist Health Studies really break their study group into well defined categories which I feel really shows well the differences of the effects of diet among people in the U.S and Canada.
https://publichealth.llu.edu/adventist-health-studies

And the results presented here I think really show what seem to be the probable outcomes for our various dietary choices. It made me really realize what path towards what probable outcomes I wanted to be on:
https://www.ncbi.nlm.nih.gov/pmc/articles/

PMC2677008/?tool=pubmed

The Nurses' Health Study (NHS) was launched in 1976 with over 121,700 nurse participants to examine the risk factors for major chronic diseases in women. https://www.nurseshealthstudy.org/

Africa is where humans and our predecessor species come from. It is where the evolution happened to design our bodies. We were there in Central Africa until about 200,000 years ago. Studying the disease rates and the nutrition of people that are still there is important to show how our bodies can function if they are given the nutrition they were evolved to consume. https://nutritionfacts.org/topics/africa/

Colon Cancer: Americans versus Africans: https://www.youtube.com/watch?v=tHngCY-JNEAo&t=107s

Rates of Alzheimers Around the World: https://nutritionfacts.org/2015/11/12/where-are-the-low-est-rates-of-alzheimers-in-the-world/

Incidence of Dementia of Black People in Nigeria versus Indiana: https://www.ncbi.nlm.nih.gov/pubmed/11176911

Austria: https://link.springer.com/article/10.1007%2Fs00508-013-0483-3

Lyon Diet Heart Study: https://www.ahajournals.org/doi/full/10.1161/01.

CIR.103.13.1823

Why Japan Lives Longer:
https://www.youtube.com/watch?v=HDUo8h29HWM

Effects of Dairy Consumption in Sweden:
https://www.care2.com/causes/does-milk-really-improve-bone-health.html

Stomach Cancer Rates:
https://www.wcrf.org/dietandcancer/cancer-trends/stomach-cancer-statistics

China Study: The **China–Cornell–Oxford Project** was a large observational study conducted throughout the 1980s in rural China, jointly funded by Cornell University, the University of Oxford, and the government of China.[1] In May 1990, The New York Times termed the study "the Grand Prix of epidemiology".
https://www.youtube.com/watch?v=LYIRwY7CFK-w&t=4774s
https://www.youtube.com/watch?v=G7rshjAZuzg

Important Studies from 2018:
https://medium.com/@Kahn642/10-important-plant-diet-vegan-research-studies-of-2018-15841245cdb7

Loma Linda:
https://www.youtube.com/watch?v=wlIPAvZospo

Diverticular Disease of the Colon: A Deficiency Disease of Western Civilization:
https://www.ncbi.nlm.nih.gov/pmc/articles/PMC1796198/

pdf/brmedj02261-0052.pdf

Pancreatic Cancer:
https://link.springer.com/article/10.1007/s10552-007-9054-0

Milk Consumption and Prostate Cancer in Western Countries:
http://www.airitilibrary.com/Publication/alDetailedMesh?docid=09647058-200709-201306270011-201306270011-467-476

The Population being Served by the Department of Defense Military Health System Provides for a Very Clear View Into the Health Challenges Facing the American Population as a Whole

Being overweight is now the leading medical reason for failing to qualify for military service. Twenty-seven percent of American young adults between the ages of 17 and 24 (i.e., over 9 million potential recruits) are unable to serve in the Armed Forces due to excess weight. This prevalence of our overweight prospective military population poses a threat to national security.

The problem makes our nation's security more expensive too. The related financial burdens are skyrocketing. Excess weight is associated with numerous costly co-morbidities, such as arthritis, hyperlipidemia, cardiac problems, chronic pain, and diabetes.

The Department of Defense (DoD) Military Health System (MHS) is one of the largest care providers in the US, serving approximately 9.2 million beneficiaries, including active-duty personnel, retirees, military spouses, and children. The annual cost associated with overweight exceeds $1 billion annually.

Moreover, 72% of veterans and a similar percentage of their beneficiaries and dependents are overweight or obese. So the military faces many of the same challenges as the general population regarding overweight and its associated conditions.

A Unique Opportunity to look at the Population of Norway that was Forced to Go on a Healthier "Diet" when the Germans Occupied:

It's interesting to look at what happened to heart attacks in Norway during World War II from 1939 to 1945 when the invading Nazis took away all of the country's meat and dairy to send to feed the German troops during the war.

The incidence of heart attacks went down until the war ended, but when they got their meat and dairy back after the war, the rate of heart attacks started climbing again. Norway Heart Attacks:
https://www.youtube.com/watch?v=HZpYkD_plPw

I was a 40 Year Old in Trouble (first wake up call):

I went in for my first big physical at age 40, never had any previous consequences from my standard American diet and activity level. It was a real wake up call. I weighed 272, my blood pressure was high, as was my cholesterol, my triglycerides were off the charts high, and my uric acid was very high. The doctor wanted me to go on three medications.

The problem as I saw it was that I was only 40! Too young to have to have one of those daily pill organizers like older people do! Plus, I hate taking medications; I'm a sensitive redhead and they always make me feel funny, and not in a ha ha good way.

Started Looking for Solutions that Didn't Involve Medications

Medications have always made me "feel funny," even in my youth, so I long ago decided I didn't like taking them. I was like a kid who decides not to eat canned green peas.

This was even after a checkup in my 20s when the doctor told me my gluttonous lifestyle was causing high levels of uric acid, which leads to extremely painful gout. I stlll wouldn't take the Allopurinal drug that he prescribed (more on how this decision came to haunt me later).

So then I was snagged by a "silver bullet" diet. The Atkins Diet -- what today's Keto Diet used to be called.

It was one of those "Hey I can do that, and, hey, it seems to make sense" decisions. It had just enough logic to help me rationalize trying it. Of course, I didn't do any research to see if it had any real science behind it or if it had any harmful side effects. (In my defense, this was long before I had easy access to an internet search engine where I could find the science and read reviews and lists of side effects.)

So after skimming through an inexpensive paperback copy of the Atkins Diet I started trying to send my body into ketosis. I bought some test strips to pee on to see when I achieved ketosis, which was when my urine turned them purple.

Well, I quickly lost about 10 pounds, but It otherwise sucked, and it sucked bad. I felt like poop, yet I couldn't poop. Bloody Hemorrhoid City here I was.

After doing some research I found out the 10 pounds I lost quickly was most likely water.......and the weight quickly came back.

According to the Mayo Clinic website talking about ketosis:
"If you suddenly and drastically cut carbs, you may experience a variety of temporary health effects, including:

- Headache
- Bad breath
- Weakness
- Muscle cramps
- Fatigue
- Skin rash
- Constipation or diarrhea

In addition, some diets restrict carbohydrate intake so much that in the long term they can result in vitamin or mineral deficiencies, bone loss and gastrointestinal disturbances and may increase risks of various chronic diseases. Emphasizing that "Chronic" means they will last a long time if not forever, just because you wanted to lose some weight.

Because low-carb diets may not provide necessary nutrients, these diets aren't recommended as a method of weight loss for preteens and high schoolers. Their growing bodies need the nutrients found in whole grains, fruits and vegetables.

Severely restricting carbohydrates to less than 0.7 ounces (20 grams) a day can result in a process called ketosis. Ketosis occurs when you don't have enough sugar (glucose) for energy, so your body breaks down stored fat, causing ketones to build up in your body. Side effects from ketosis can include nausea, headache, mental and physical fatigue, and bad breath.

It's not clear if a low-carb diet poses long-term health risks; most studies have lasted less than a year, too short a period to calculate long-term impacts and didn't examine. Some health experts believe that if you eat large amounts of fat and protein from animal sources, your risk of heart disease or certain cancers may actually increase.

If you follow a low-carbohydrate diet that's higher in fat and possibly higher in protein, it's important to choose foods with healthy unsaturated fats and healthy proteins. Limit foods containing saturated and trans fats, such as meat, high-fat dairy products, and processed crackers and pastries.

The Keto Diet Debunked:
https://www.youtube.com/watch?v=MzHLAqyO7PQ

Many consider Dr. Atkins to be a "snake oil" salesman. He made millions yet he never spent a dime to test his diet theory to see if it worked or was safe. But he didn't need to because he was telling a lot of people what they wanted to hear. There is a substantial segment of the "health advice" industry that seems to cater to people who want to justify their bad habits.

Harvard researchers have determined that low carb diets increase the chances of many diseases, and all cause mortality, so I really wish I had known this about low carb diets before I tried it:
https://www.youtube.com/watch?v=bmDUnFd6UX4

Former President of the American College of Cardiology says that No One Should do the Keto Diet:
https://bigthink.com/stephen-johnson/no-one-should-be-doing-the-ketogenic-diet-says-former-president-of-the-american-college-of-cardiology

Silver Bullets ...

Like many people, I was looking for the "silver bullets" that were going to take care of everything without much effort ... if I ate oat bran, drank red wine, took fish oil pills, cut out gluten, took supplements, cut out carbs and even forced my body into ketosis, drank more water, switched to antibiotic free and/or free range animals, etc.

Since my very bad checkup at age 40, I have been looking for non-medication solutions. What I have learned over the last 20 some years of looking for them is:
- There are no silver bullets that work for very long.
- There are a lot of people out there trying to sell things and claiming they have silver bullets.
- These sellers have a huge open market of people looking for an instant or relatively quick easy fix to problems.
- Even the "legitimate" medical industry in many ways is also selling fixes, some short term, but usually very much to the benefit of shareholders, they are very long term fixes (i.e. you will take statins your whole life once prescribed).

History of "Silver Bullets"... per the website Health. com

1727 - The Avoiding Swamps Diet, Thomas Short observed that overweight people live near swamps. So the solution was to move away from them.

1820 - Lord Byron popularized a vinegar and water diet.

1864 - William Banting's "Letter on Corpulence," likely was the first diet book ever published. Mr. Banting was an overweight undertaker, wrote his book to espouse his success after replacing an excessive intake of bread, sugar and potatoes with mostly meat, fish and vegetables. (I guess I am espousing my health successes with this book)

1925 - Lucky Strike cigs says: "reach for a Lucky instead of a sweet."

1930s - Grapefruit Diet, also known as the Hollywood Diet.

1941 - Lemonade Diet or "Master Cleanse."

1950s - Cabbage Soup Diet.

1950s - Apple Cider Vinegar Diet (rebirth of Lord Byron's Diet).

1950s - Tapeworm Diet.

1960s - The Drinking Man's Diet.

1963 - Weight Watchers begins (this one actually has some benefit).

1960s - Weight Loss Chocolates called "Ayds."

1969 - Jazzercise Founded.

1970 - Sleeping Beauty Diet, made famous by Elvis (involving sedation).

1970s - Andy Warhol Diet - order food you don't really like so you don't eat very much, then have it packaged to go so you can give it to a homeless person on your walk home.

1975 - The Cookie Diet.

1976 - The Last Chance Diet (basically a meat smoothie).

1977 - Slim-Fast Diet.

1978 - The Complete Scarsdale Medical Diet.

1979 - Dexatrim®, a diet drug containing phenylpropanolamine (PPA), appears on drugstore shelves. Its formula changes after PPA is linked to an increased risk of stroke in 2000

1982 - Jane Fonda releases her first Aerobics video tape and coined the phrase: "No Pain, No Gain."

1983 - Jazzercise is now in all 50 states.

1985 - Fit for Life Diet.

1992 - Dr. Atkins' New Diet Revolution is published.

1994 - Nutrition Labeling Act requires information on packaged food.

1995 - The Zone Diet.

2000 - Macrobiotic Diet.

2003 - The South Beach Diet.

2003 - Seven Day Color Diet.

2004 - Ephedra banned due to heart attack risk.

2004 – "The Biggest Loser" reality show begins.

2006 - Beyoncé uses The Master Cleanse.

2007 - "Alli"® an OTC drug that stops absorption of food by the body introduced.

2010 - Jennifer Hudson loses 80 pounds on Weight Watchers.

2011 - The HCG Diet, which combines a fertility drug with a strict 500- to 800-calorie-a-day regimen.

2012 - Jessica Simpson loses 60 pounds of baby weight on Weight Watchers.

2013 - Cotton Ball Diet.

2013 - Victoria Beckham tweeted about the Alkaline Diet.

2018/2019 – Currently the 2 popular diets are the Paleo and the Keto diets, or packaged variations like the Whole 30 diet.

So Easy to Get Overwhelmed
by Messages

There is so much information flow out there that I was overwhelmed and confused for a long time but I kept slogging through it, mainly because even though I had made improvements in some areas I still wasn't completely satisfied with the way I felt physically or the way I felt about the way I looked when I looked in the mirror.

There are so many ideas and products being sold and many ideas that can conflict and confuse.

But there is also information available that has been developed, gathered, and discovered using legitimate scientific methods.

The way in which most people gain their information is very casual and almost random. It isn't always from sources that are seeking to deliver the facts or truth, but instead from stories with headlines that will catch people's attention and get them to watch a show or to pick up printed material.

An example is Studies Showing Saturated Fat like Butter

is OK:
https://www.youtube.com/watch?v=OIZaZq5lUew

Many official looking legitimate sounding entities are distributing "news" and information that doesn't have your
best interests at heart. It's merely designed to make money
for themselves and helps you justify complacency by continuing your well established habits.

The Dairy Industry for instance has been putting out messages to try and scare people about drinking nondairy
milks such as soy:
https://www.youtube.com/watch?v=0GiXZam27Q4

We all wish there were "Silver Bullets" that would be easy
to take and would allow us to continue to eat, drink and
smoke anything. I know I was looking for it, and I tried a
number of them.

One of the main lessons I have learned over my twenty
year journey is that "Diets Do Not Work"! They are not
sustainable. Anyway, soon there will be a new diet on next
month's magazines that will cause many people to switch
to the next best thing.

Desires Controlled by the Food Industry:
https://www.youtube.com/watch?v=KtdgjvO5qVM

Second Wake Up Call (a very very painful one 18 years ago):

I woke up to the light weight of the sheet causing severe pain to my big toe.

It was a searing, sharp, intense pain—like fire. I wanted to cut my big toe off with a hatchet, because it wouldn't have hurt as much.

I had the "Disease of Kings," also known as gout. It affects 1 out of 100 people and 5 out of 100 men over the age of 65. But I was only 43.

It is a lifestyle disease from eating rich foods. Hence the name Disease of Kings because in the days of old, only the rich people could afford foods it's caused by. Paupers and peasants did not get gout.

Being a glutton, as I am, I am the poster child for the affliction. This is something I am not very proud of, but it did get me to refocus my efforts on trying to have a healthier lifestyle, eating better and getting some exercise. I still have never taken drugs for gout and have chosen to manage it with diet and exercise.

Not always successfully I might add, but it has kept me vigilant which I think has been a good thing for me for the long term. It has enabled me to truly overcome it rather than just medicating, (bandaging) it and continuing to eat badly.

It has kept me from being a fat slob couch potato because it hurts too much. Otherwise I would most likely be over 300 pounds. I maxed out at 272 at age 40, and am now down to 208 at age 61. I'm hoping to get down to 200—my goal—but I'm going to have to start restricting calories and/or getting some exercise to get there.

Unfortunately I like bread too much, both traditional and liquid (beer).

The Horror of Observing
Parents Suffer

L ooking back, it's kind of amazing to realize what we used to accept as "normal." As kids (my two sisters and I), we watched both our parents smoke; father heavily and mother regularly. Smoke was everywhere. We three little kids in the backseat of a smoke-filled car was "normal;" it was the 1960s.

So it was also "normal" when, as a kid, we would make ashtrays for our parents during grade school arts and crafts.

For Father's Day, or for his birthday, we would buy Dad smoking accessories as gifts ... or cigars or pipe tobacco. It was "normal". Once shopping malls came along there was a store called the "Tinder Box" where we used to go buy gifts that contributed to our father's early death.

At some point in the 1960s, despite the tobacco company denials, the anti-smoking campaigns began. In school they taught us about the dangers, and posters with a particularly scary looking woman smoking, caused us kids to become "anti-smoking activists." We tried to tell our parents what we learned, and I remember that not going over so well.

Anti-Smoking Poster we saw in school:
https://images.app.goo.gl/kmmG7W5BGfYcgGC76

Already addicted to tobacco, they didn't want to hear the truth.

Our father either didn't know or chose to ignore the science that was becoming available in the 1950s and 60s about the effects of tobacco use on the human body.

Dad, for as long as I can ever remember, woke up each morning hacking and coughing and spitting out mucus and blowing his nose. We would hear this from under our covers as it sounded like dad was going to cough a lung out.

It was the "normal" sound of the morning until we heard the front door close and the truck start and drive off. Actually he coughed so much and so loud we could hear him cough and spit all the way out to the truck in the driveway. It was "normal" for him, and for us.

Dad said they gave them all free cigarettes when he was in the Marine Corps in the early 1950s, telling the soldiers that cigarettes would help keep them alert. He told me this looking up sadly from a hospital bed.

His 59th year he was in and out of several Veterans Administration Hospitals for numerous procedures including having his chest opened up and half of one of his lungs cut out, and then lots of radiation therapy, which he said really hurt. Hurt to swallow, burned, hurt to breathe.

Over the last 6 months of Dad's life, I was called by the nurses in his ward numerous times to tell me to come to say goodbye as they did not expect him to make it through the night. I jumped in my car and drove the 5 hours to Iowa City and then, after he was transferred, the 4 hours to Danville where I would spend a number of hours with him each time.

Towards the end, he couldn't really say much because he was gasping for air and he was so loaded up on morphine, but I would stand there and look into the eyes of a drowning man helpless to do anything for him.

One time a nurse said that his heart seemed so strong which is why he did not die as they had predicted. Finally, a nurse told me they were giving him massive doses of acetaminophen to control his run away fever and that usually kills about anyone after a week. She was right.

Our once healthy, big and strong father, whose picture in his Marine Corp sergeant's uniform made him kind of look like John Wayne, died a horrible painful suffering death at age 60 after drowning and gasping for air and sweating in his hospital bed for months.

As I write this I am looking at my father's death certificate which says he died of "Squamous Cell Cancer of Lung" at 11:30 PM at the Danville V.A. hospital. The day after my 34th birthday, and 2 months after his 60th. He was alone, but so out of it from the fever and the morphine, as I had seen him that way a couple of days before then when I last saw him alive.

Whatever the "medical condition" was called was kind of irrelevant. The cause of Dad's early death was absorbing something on a regular basis that his body was never designed to process. The human body evolved from millions of years ago to hundreds of thousands of years ago and there was no tobacco use influencing the genetic changes in the evolutionary process.

Tobacco has been growing wild in the Americas for nearly **8,000 years**. Around **2,000 years** ago tobacco began to be chewed and smoked during cultural or religious ceremonies and events by the indigenous peoples of North America.

People of European descent, like my father, were first introduced to tobacco use by the Spanish explorers and settlers in 1528. The chemical compounds in tobacco are not anything the human body was engineered by evolution to process properly.

As scientific study has proven, tobacco causes our natural processes to be disrupted and our cell regeneration processes to mutate into tumors and cancer cells which often multiply and spread.

Our dad told me he started smoking at age 15, which would have been 1946 -- only 418 years after Europeans started smoking, little time for any evolutionary adaptation.

So am I passionate about keeping myself from suffering

and dying like my dad did at the end of his life? Yes and so almost daily for two years now I have been plowing into the internet and books to get down past the "noise" created by then the tobacco and now the food industries and into the actual science about the effects of what we take into our bodies.

What I have learned is: We are what we absorb.

Cigarettes contain more than 4000 chemicals, of which 40 are known carcinogens and 400 more are known toxins. But let's just focus on one chemical, Benzene, which is the compound that is most likely to cause leukemia (blood cancer) in humans. This carcinogen has been well known in the scientific literature since the 1950s.

A compound that is one of the most basic petrochemicals and is present in crude oil, Benzene is commonly used in gasoline and pesticides. Smoking causes almost half of benzene exposure to humans.

Anemia, genetic damage and excessive bleeding are also ailments that can be caused by this compound, yet some 37,000,000 people in the US still inhale and absorb it through their cigarettes every day.

Dad absorbed some nasty stuff and paid the price so I am working to learn what I can absorb, and not absorb, to promote longevity and defer pain and suffering.

Besides lung diseases, there seem to be multiple epidemics of diseases that I don't remember people talking about when I was a kid. So many people seem to be overweight and have mis-shaped bodies. I was in the obese zone of BMI (body mass index) before I started on this path, but not anymore.

The first reports of the Surgeon General about smoking came in 1964. In 1965 Congress put warnings on cigarettes. In 1969 cigarette ads were banned on radio and TV, effective September 1970. My father died from smoking in November 1991. Looking back, the science was being published pretty regularly in the 1950s, but it took a while for the information to get out and become widely accepted.

One day I realized my father and I seemed to be on a parallel track with nutrition. There is science about nutrition out there now, just like there was about tobacco use in the 1950s.

But just like with tobacco use, people can be uninformed, or uncaring about it, choose to ignore it, or use the power of rationalization to not do anything about it. And industry funded "studies" and "messages" about those studies have proven to be very powerful at aiding our rationalizations. The tobacco industry wrote the playbook on how to confuse the issue and keep people using their products, despite the science.

How Smoking in the 1950s is like eating industrial food today:
https://nutritionfacts.org/video/how-smoking-in-the-50s-is-like-eating-today/

But I very much believe in personal choice. Each person has a right to do what they want to with their one life. But for my kids and friends, please at least read and thoughtfully consider what I am trying to present here. **Many "Lifestyle" diseases that come from what we ingest and absorb are devastating**. I've seen it up close and personal. Please don't go down that path voluntarily.

The list of diseases caused by "lifestyle and nutrition" choices just goes on and on: heart disease, various cancers, diabetes, Parkinson's, high blood pressure, stroke, Alzheimer's, ALS, bowel problems, and so many more.

In my opinion, the Surgeon General is unlikely to issue a warning for foods like they did for cigarettes. Food production and farming are important industries in every state of the union and so Congress is heavily influenced by them. Tobacco is only important in a handful of states and didn't have the power to stop the Surgeon General, even though they tried.

If you were in high school or college in the 50s or 60s and someone offered you a cigarette and you turned it down citing health reasons, you were probably socially derided or teased and called a "square" or a "goody two shoes" or a "momma's boy."

I used to assume that cigarette smoking mostly affected and damaged the lungs directly, which they do of course, but the absorption of hydrocarbons, some of them known to be highly carcinogenic (think Benzene), into the bone marrow, has significant effects as well.

Our bone marrow is where our red blood cells are produced and the majority of our white blood cells, and according to the NIeH other important cells that help us to heal ourselves:

> "*Cigarette smoking is known for its deleterious effect on many systems and organs. It is linked to a significant decrease in bone marrow concentration of mesenchymal stem cells. This reduced cell population may contribute to the reduced regenerative capacity of smokers, with potentially important implications for physiological maintenance and repair in the musculoskeletal system.*"

Watching Mom Suffer in a Hospital Bed

Mom didn't smoke as much as Dad, but she didn't avoid the consequences either. 2018 was like 1991 all over again.

It almost killed me looking down at her so sick, looking into those sad and helpless eyes. She was weak, angry, and had some form of dementia setting in.

What also made me crazy was that in 2018, with all the science that is available, the hospital and the rehab center were feeding her the things that probably got her there in the first place:

- Sausage and gravy
- Eggs and cheese
- Greasy beef chili
- Hamburger meat
- Lots of meat and fatty foods

I had to ask for fruit to be served every meal.

Alzheimer's Disease Rates around the World:
https://www.youtube.com/watch?v=2_l-dqPyD0w&t=31s

Look at All the Deformed Bodies

Processed food, and the obesity that comes with it has deformed the natural shape of the human body. I don't remember people looking like this 50 years ago when I was a kid, with enormous butts, hips, and distended bellies, huge saddlebags on their thighs, and big jowls hanging from their chins and necks. And we have exported it to most parts of the world so they can enjoy the same lifestyle diseases that are epidemic here.

I am so happy that my body has gone back towards my natural shape and I am now no longer in the obese range for BMI. I would have an even better shape if I stopped drinking so much beer and wine, so I'm not claiming dietary perfection. Just major, major improvement.
https://www.plantbasednews.org/opinion/10-mind-blowing-vegan-transformations

I have been to Europe many times both for business and pleasure and when I look around, it is hard to find people with such deformed bodies as we have here in the U.S. When I do see them they turn out to be from the U.S.

Granny from Missouri

My parents bought an acre of land from my mom's parents to build a house the year after I was born, so I grew up spending a lot of time with my maternal grandparents.

They were both self-employed, working from the home property. Granny raised a huge garden, had a small vineyard of concord grapes, and sold produce along the "hard road", canned and froze anything and everything for home consumption, and there were 4 rental properties on the five acres that she mostly maintained.

The only time I ever saw her sit still was early each morning when I was having my corn flakes. She would come over to try and talk to my mom.

But when I was 13, they found Granny dead on her kitchen linoleum having had some sudden life ending event. She was a young 67 with hardly any gray hair.

It was quite a shock because of all our grandparents she was the most active. She was the strongest and was seemingly tireless—she never stopped moving, working and doing something productive.

But I can still remember the kitchen drawer full of pill bottles and supplements right next to her silverware drawer, the bacon grease jar that was always on the stove and the softened butter stick that was on a plate in the cupboard ready to be slathered on biscuits or toast.

I never saw Granny cook with anything other than bacon grease, margarine or Crisco (the softened butter was just for the table). God only knows what took her, the pills or the saturated or trans fats. But the good thing is Granny went fast and did not suffer for long.

Toxins

Let's talk about the science of toxins—how they get into the body and what they cause to happen, and then how the body gets rid of them.

Remember that the human body has about a trillion cells (that is a million million,) and most of those cells regenerate about every 100 days. The cell regeneration process can either be:

1. Fed with good biological inputs that support the over 1000 metabolic functions in the human body.
2. Starved by not getting enough inputs.
3. Messed with by molecules that the body did not evolve to process, some of which can be classified as Toxins.

It's hard to wrap one's head around the whole cell-regeneration thing, but consider that much of the dust around your home is dead skin cells that have flaked off our bodies from the cell regeneration process.

After about 10 years our mattresses are supposedly full of dead skin cells and dust mites from the same process. So you can look at your arms and think not much is really happening, but yeah, it is happening, all through our bodies.

Think about the chemical compounds(many of them toxins) from tobacco use being absorbed and messing with cell regeneration.

One of my favorite sayings has always been, "We are what we eat", but since studying the biochemistry of the science of nutrition my new favorite saying is: "We are what we absorb."

This is because what we absorb is what our cells have available to regenerate themselves with. So absorption of good nutrients as well as proper transport to the cells are both important, and are critical for efficiently removing toxins too.

You've heard the saying, "Garbage in, garbage out." Consider the photos in the links below: identical twins, so they have the same genetic makeup, but one of them smokes and one does not.
https://www.cnn.com/2013/10/31/health/smoking-aging-identical-twins/index.html

This is what toxins can do to your body.

By now, most people understand and accept that smoking tobacco puts toxins into our bodies, but where do toxins come from in our food? Well consider things like high fructose corn syrup, aspartame, sucralose, pesticides, fungicides, herbicides and other toxins that get into our air, water and food and then get absorbed into our bodies.

Jim Stoecker

And since we are pretty much at the top of the food chain, we ingest all the toxins that were eaten and absorbed by all the animals we eat which multiplies toxins by a process called bioaccumulation.

So if a cow eats tons of grass and corn that has been sprayed with chemicals, then over time those toxins accumulate in the flesh of the cow, and then it gets put on your plate as that big juicy hamburger.

So even if the lettuce and tomato on the burger have been sprayed by chemicals, they have a whole lot less toxins because they were only sprayed once, where the cow ate tons of food sprayed with toxins.

Toxins are dose dependent meaning in small doses they may not cause harm but larger doses can cross a line and cause harm.

The news is filled with warnings that certain fish, like swordfish, that eat lots of smaller fish, who in turn have eaten many even smaller fish, have bio-accumulated high levels of toxins like mercury.
https://www.canada.ca/en/environment-climate-change/services/pollutants/mercury-environment/health-concerns/food-chain.html

The good news is that our bodies evolved to dispose of toxins because we developed and evolved in very close proximity with, and consuming, naturally occuring toxins.

There are a lot of naturally occurring toxins in our world, other things like plants also evolved to survive and they may have things toxic to bugs that are also mildly toxic to humans and so the body has processes to get those out of our systems. We mostly pee and poop them out.

But the fiber we eat is very important to help the process.

Bile is one of the main ways the body processes toxins safely out of our bodies, and fiber is very important to carrying these toxic bile salts out of our digestive tracts and into the toilet bowl. **Having a sufficient amount of fiber in our diets to grab on to the toxic bile excretion and get it out of us is critical to our survival.**

What binds to bile the best:
https://www.youtube.com/watch?v=AAHl20vJqqQ

If we don't eat enough fiber to carry the stuff out then our intestines re-absorb the toxins so they are recirculated through our bodily systems.

I made up this acronym: BBaBBa - Beets Best at Bile Binding Ability.

I don't think anyone needs to know anything about science to understand that toxins recirculating through our bodies cannot be a good thing.

Get the Lead Out:
https://www.youtube.com/watch?v=ahj6GLvl7oQ

Can Saunas help detoxify the body?
https://www.youtube.com/watch?v=ypkjUy_jghQ

Deep Frying to Make Toxins:
https://www.youtube.com/watch?v=i6vdycYq3SI

Lighten Your Toxic Load
In general, to minimize your exposure to toxins, it's a good idea to switch from personal care products containing harmful ingredients, to ones that are more natural. Check ingredients on labels and avoid the following:

Acrylates
Aluminum
Formaldehyde
Fragrance
Oxybenzone
Parabens
Phthalates
Polyethylene glycols
Triclosan
Lead

What goes on your body, goes in your body.

Blood Flow is So Important!!!

In addition to what we absorb, nutrients and cells get transported everywhere in the body by the blood flow where they create the proper environment for cell regeneration.

When it comes to taking care of your cardiovascular system little to no attention is typically given to your endothelial cells. Almost all of the attention goes to your heart or your arteries and veins. Yet, more and more research is showing that the health of your heart, arteries, veins and all of your cardiovascular system is dependent upon the health of your endothelial cells.

What are Endothelial Cells?

Endothelial cells are the thin layer of cells that line the interior surface of all blood vessels. It is sometimes referred to as the endothelium. It's important to note that these cells line the entire circulatory system from the heart all the way down to the smallest capillary.

When added up, the volume of these endothelial cells would cover the surface area of 8 tennis courts and weigh as much as the liver. That's amazing since the endotheli-um is only one cell thick and can't be seen by the human eye.

The endothelium's gate-keeping role varies for each organ system. For example, in the brain and retina the endothe-lial cells are tightly linked together to create a barrier that only allows selective molecules to pass through it. In the liver, spleen and bone marrow, the endothelial cells are loosely linked allowing for cellular trafficking between these intercellular gaps.

However, in the kidneys, endocrine glands and intestinal villi, the endothelial cells have a different type of selective permeability to allow for efficient filtering, secretion and absorption based on that organ's function.

Two critical functions I want to highlight are the endothe-lium's role in angiogenesis and atherosclerosis. Angiogen-esis is the formation of new capillaries. This function is ex-tremely important in wound healing.

It also plays a significant role in muscle creation and in the heart's ability to develop collateral vessels. These col-lateral vessels can help lessen the impact of a blood vessel blockage in the heart by providing alternative routes for blood flow.

The endothelium also plays a leading role in atheroscler-sis or hardening of the arteries. It does this by providing a smooth surface that inhibits platelet adhesion and clotting. It also tries to inhibit foreign substances from adhering to its cellular wall which can lead to plaque formations.

Large molecules like cholesterol and/or toxic substances like nicotine, damage the intercellular junctions between the endothelial cells allowing deposits to build up.

This causes the smooth and flexible lining of your blood vessels to become rough and hard, and hence the term hardening of the arteries. As this process continues over time, the deposits or plaques become larger which narrows the interior of the blood vessel making it harder for blood to pass through.

This increases resistance to blood flow which can cause your blood pressure to increase. The following contributing factors can cause the endothelium to lose its ability to prevent these formations: smoking, diabetes, hyperlipidemia, hypertension or high blood pressure, and inflammation. Elevated homocysteine levels have also been associated with premature atherosclerosis.

Atherosclerosis was once thought to be irreversible but new studies clearly show that when the proper biochemical environment is provided the injured endothelium can return to its undamaged state.

In 1998 the Nobel Prize in medicine was awarded to 3 Americans who identified what they called "the atom" of cardiovascular health—a tiny molecule called nitric oxide.

Symbol "NO"—as it is known by chemists—is produced by the body specifically to help keep arteries and veins free of the plaque that causes stroke and to maintain normal blood pressure by relaxing the arteries, and regulating the rate of blood flow, which helps prevent coronaries. Nitric oxide (NO) is the body's natural cardiovascular wonder drug.

These discoveries—the role of the endothelium, and the benefits of nitric oxide are great news for those who struggle with heart disease—or would like to make sure they don't.

Foods High in Nitric Oxide:
https://www.livestrong.com/article/465685-list-of-foods-high-in-nitric-oxide/

To give this issue about blood flow even more credibility, let me introduce Dr. Caldwell Esselstyn from the Cleveland Clinic. As you may know, the Cleveland Clinic has long been considered the leader in cardiovascular medicine. It publishes the peer-reviewed journal *Cleveland Clinic Journal of Medicine.*

Watch what he has to say in this 14 minute video about the heart, blood flow, and Nitric Oxide.
https://www.youtube.com/watch?v=EqKNfyUPzoU

Blood flow to every cell of your body with the proper nutrients is so important

Where do You Get Your Protein?

Almost without exception, like pulling a gun quickly to defend themselves, the most common question I get about my science based way of nutrition is, where do you get your protein? I try to be patient, but actually from what I have learned about the science, it would be hard NOT to get "enough" protein.

It's in nearly everything natural that we eat. I'm talking about plants here—not the chemically created, processed and doesn't happen to contain animal by products junk food. But even most of those thngs have some protein too, it is everywhere.

Consider for example, the Gorilla, our genetic cousin, which shares 97% of our DNA, and which is estimated to be about 30 times stronger than the average human, and is just ripped with solid muscle, well, they eat fruits and leaves. So they get plenty of protein obviously to make all that muscle.

Or the Ox, another very muscular mammal that eats grass, and gets plenty of protein to build all that muscle.

Or consider human breast milk which is the perfect food

for humans to consume during the period of our lives when we are growing and developing the fastest. Human breast milk has much less protein in it than bovine breast milk.

Getting protein is simply not a problem. But the question does illustrate the lack of current true nutritional information in the general public.

Blood Test Results on Protein Levels:
https://www.youtube.com/watch?v=xGd8Mw9NaI4

The China Study is a comprehensive collection of scientific information about nutrition and covers a lot about protein.
https://www.youtube.com/watch?v=G7rshjAZuzg

I find it ironic that many people have such an emotional reaction as if they are concerned for me about, "Where do I get my Protein" when there are virtually no reported cases of any kind of protein deficiency in the US.

Yet these same people would have no concern about the overwhelming statistics about my chances of heart disease if they were sitting with me watching me eat a half pound bacon, cheese burger, a pound of french fries and a gallon of Coke® or beer.

I've seen horrified looks on people's faces when I tell them I eat fruits, veggies, leaves and maybe some tofu, but there probably would be no adverse reaction if I told them I ate 20 deep fried chicken wings.

Some people say "yuck" if I mention I eat tofu, but they have no problem eating the flesh of dead animals that spent most of their miserable lives standing or laying down, breathing and eating in their own filth. I

n such disgusting conditions they have to be regularly fed antibiotics to keep them alive until they are chopped up in such a way that the flesh is contaminated with the bacteria from their intestines such that the flesh has to be handled like hazardous waste.
https://www.brendadavisrd.com/legumes-vs-meat/

I have enjoyed pretty much completely plant based nutrition now for over 2 years and my recent blood test showed my protein at the high end of the acceptable range.

Where are You Going to Get Your New Kidneys?

Chronic kidney disease doubled from 1990 to 2010 and one in eight of us now has chronic kidney disease, and to make matters even more concerning, three quarters of those people don't even know they have it.

All that "high quality protein" as some people like to call it, is putting a lot of stress on our delicate essential kidneys and their ability to function properly.
https://www.youtube.com/watch?v=58PBof9oUK8

S.O.S. = Salt. Oil. Sugar. The way many people regularly ingest these processed substances also puts a lot of stress on our kidneys both directly and when they end up with diabetes. I see dialysis clinic storefronts pretty much everywhere I drive these days. Ever see the arms of someone who goes in for dialysis?

Can We Get All the Nutrients We Need Without Eating Animals?

The Position of the American Dietetic Association and the Dietitians of Canada is that:

"Well-planned vegan and other types of vegetarian diets are appropriate for all stages of the life cycle, including during pregnancy, lactation, infancy, childhood, and adolescence. Vegetarian diets offer a number of nutritional benefits, including lower levels of saturated fat, cholesterol, and animal protein as well as higher levels of carbohydrates, fiber, magnesium, potassium, folate, and antioxidants such as vitamins C and E and phytochemicals. Vegetarians have been reported to have lower body mass indices than non-vegetarians, as well as lower rates of death from ischemic heart disease; vegetarians also show lower blood cholesterol levels; lower blood pressure; and lower rates of hypertension, type 2 diabetes, and prostate and colon cancer."

How Much Protein Do We Need?

Here is a calculator that can give you a pretty good idea. The results may surprise you.

This tool will calculate daily nutrient recommendations based on the Dietary Reference Intakes (DRIs) established by the Health and Medicine Division of the National Academies of Sciences, Engineering and Medicine.

The data represents the most current scientific knowledge on nutrient needs however individual requirements may be higher or lower than DRI recommendations.

By entering height, weight, age, and activity level, you will generate a report of: Body Mass Index, estimated daily calorie needs in addition to the recommended intakes of macronutrients, vitamins, and minerals based on DRI data. https://fnic.nal.usda.gov/fnic/dri-calculator/

How is Your Sleep

The science of this one is huge for me because I need motivation to drink less alcohol and cut out midnight snacks.
https://getpocket.com/explore/item/this-is-what-your-overactive-brain-needs-to-get-a-good-night-s-sleep?utm_source=pocket-newtab

I sleep much better now and I wake up with great energy!

Laws versus Beliefs

There are natural laws that are unavoidable—like gravity, or the effects of the sun on unprotected skin. And there are beliefs, which may or may not line up with natural laws. The problems come when we confuse laws with beliefs.

You may believe gravity doesn't apply to you, but if you jump off a cliff, it will catch up with you. We may remain blissfully ignorant of natural laws if we haven't tried to break them, and intellectual knowledge of them may not change our actions. But we will always act in concert with what we believe. In the best case scenarios, we align the two.

It isn't easy to open up the mind to examine one's beliefs to see how they might be in conflict with natural laws. But it can be dangerous and painful to ignore this information. https://nutritionfacts.org/topics/bacon/

The "Oh It's Genetic it Runs in My Family" Rationalization

I am a redhead with blue eyes which makes me a "one percenter". Genetically speaking, those with my coloring make up only one percent of the population.

So having been a kid before they invented sunscreen with SPF factors I have some up close and painfully personal experience with sunburns, and I could easily blame genetics.

In fact, I have heard many people rationalize their troubles by using the genetic predisposition argument. You know like when they say that obesity runs in my family, or my mom had breast cancer or polyps in her colon so I guess I will too—it is just the deck of cards I was dealt. In doing this they absolve themselves of responsibility, resigned to their "fate" as they consume another rasher of bacon and cheesy potatoes.

According to dermatologist Neal Schultz, M.D., host of DermTV, "At the root of it, a sunburn is damage—and ultimately, death—to some of the cells of the epidermis layer of the skin." In technical terms, "ultraviolet damage causes **free radical production and oxidative stress, which caus-**

es DNA damage," This then "causes a cascade of different tiers of chemical and cellular mediators of inflammation and damage."

In recognizable terms: inflammation is the redness, swelling, and sensation of discomfort (or burning) that you get with a sunburn. And the induced cell death and the concomitant inflammation are responsible for the peeling skin several days after your initial burn."

OK, I think we can all easily see that I as a red haired blue eyed person, have the genetic predisposition to easily sunburn and to get really bad sunburns. But did the genetic predisposition cause the sunburn and damage to my skin? No, putting my skin cells in an environment of exposing myself to the sun is what caused the damage to the skin.

So please remember this concept: **"Genetics may have loaded the gun, but they didn't pull the trigger."**

In more scientific terms: "Yes you may have certain types of genes, but the environment you provide for them to live in and regenerate in is what causes them to express themselves in different ways both good and bad."

Let's listen to some research about sun exposure, oxidative damage, and the consumption of antioxidants and or alcohol......Preventing Skin Cancer from the Inside Out: https://www.youtube.com/watch?v=YvlBppBSKZM

Cruising Observations:

I recently went on a cruise, and it was very motivational regarding my new way of eating. I noticed many fellow cruisers waddled vs. walking. And watching what people were eating in the buffet area, it was so obvious why some people were waddling, or had difficulty walking, or had knee braces.

They were collapsing under their own weight. The piles of bacon and sausages on their plates showed what was contributing to the excess weight.

I talked to a lady on the cruise who asked me about my book; her response was at 65 she was going to eat whatever she wanted in order to live her life and not worry about what she ate all the time.

She disclosed she was on medications for cholesterol and anxiety attacks. She was overweight and carried a lot of loose skin around her neck. Of course her lifestyle choices are her right to make, but I couldn't help feeling they were short sighted.

Then one morning I watched as a morbidly obese woman, with a t-shirt that read: "Giving Children with Cancer a

Fighting Chance", was eating breakfast sausage links like they were French fries. All I could think was, "You are giving cancer a fighting chance in your own body by the way you are eating."

Overall, rather than being "tempted" by the food on the cruise, I was very motivated to eat well by what seemed like a higher than average percentage of people who were morbidly obese.

The head chef on the cruise was from India, so they actually had some great vegetarian and even vegan dishes available, in addition to all the great fruits and veggies on the menus and at the buffets.

I had choices each morning at the buffet on the cruise ship. Did I want to eat things that will help my body try to function properly? Or eat the eggs benedict and other things that would require me to take pills to trick my body into processing things differently?

It was a mental game, and that morning I won and I felt great—I ate spinach and mushrooms from the omelet bar with low sodium soy sauce, and ate roasted potatoes with tabasco, and then fresh fruit: melon, berries, apricots and pears.

I think about how few minutes if not seconds of pleasure I get when I eat, chew and swallow certain foods, and then possibly the misery at the end of my life they may cause me.

One favorite saying I have heard is:

Jim Stoecker

"A Minute on the Lips, and a Lifetime on the Hips".

Another saying with a good reminder is:
"The Fat You Eat is the Fat You Wear."

Stalking Unsuspecting Women at the Grocery Store:

I didn't mean for it to start out that way, it just sort of happened when I noticed something.....

So I was walking through the store, and was headed in a direction that took me near the meat section when I noticed a lady struggling. She was seated in one of those motorized carts they keep plugged in and charging near the front of the store.

But she was trying to reach into one of the refrigerated display cases trying to lift a big piece of beef that looked like a roast, out of the case and into her cart. Being the former boy scout I am, I asked if she needed help.

In a very wheezing voice that sounded like she was about to drown in her own saliva, she said yes, and thank you so much. I would guess this woman was in her late 50s or early 60s.

I lifted the huge piece of cellophane wrapped beef into her cart and I noticed she already had sausages, ham, and some white bread in her cart. I told her she was welcome and went on my way to the freezer section to look for some sprouted grain bread, which is supposed to be healthier.

At the freezer case ahead of me was a lady in yoga pants with a very nice shape. When she turned around I could see she was also in her 50s or 60s, so this gave me an idea for my own study.

For the next hour I pretended to shop, but I loitered in a place where I could see both the meat section and the frozen "health foods" section, the section with veggie burgers, fake breakfast sausages, frozen gluten free products etc. My study was certainly subjective and not very scientific, but it was during a random period of time, about from 2 to 3 pm.

There were certainly a lot more people shopping for meat than for "health foods", but everyone who was shopping for meat did not look very healthy. Many had trouble walking, all looked overweight, and the color of their skin was not good. As a contrast, the people looking in the health food section all seemed to be walking well and were not as overweight as the others.

So now whenever I go to the store I always look to see who is buying meat and who is say in the organic produce section. And for many months now the results have been consistent. My personal conclusion from this observation is that people who eat a lot of meat are not healthy.

Our Ancestors Ate Meat, So Should We?:
https://www.youtube.com/watch?v=x8o6q294vXU

Carcinogens in Meat:
https://www.youtube.com/watch?v=PsZ0qdYtQBo

Is Organic Meat less Carcinogenic?:
https://www.youtube.com/watch?v=aSHv5vDi3Is

Meat a Risk Factor for Diabetes:
https://www.youtube.com/watch?v=6t4tBmbPko8

Did Meat Help our Ancestors to Become Humans?:
https://www.youtube.com/watch?v=cgmfRUwqGy4

Oh My this Obese Woman is Hard to Watch, but pay attention to what they purchase:
https://www.youtube.com/watch?v=zPlAyrrVdF8

Grossing myself out has been a very effective strategy in helping me change my consumption:

I used to go to lunch with a guy I did business with, and he had his favorite spots, so off we went. Well this was back in my eating anything that wasn't nailed down days, and a couple of these places had real good hamburgers, and I loved burgers.

After a while I noticed he never ordered a burger and so I asked him why. His answer was that hamburgers had ground into them all the gristle and fat that he trimmed off and didn't want to eat when he was served a steak. That helped me wean myself off of burgers way back in the days when I first went vegetarian and lost almost 40 pounds.

Definition of Gristle: cartilage, especially when found as tough, inedible tissue in meat (inedible until they grind it up into your burger).

I use thoughts like that today to keep myself from wanting some of the foods I used to eat. Like sausage, I used to love pork sausage. Sausage pizza was my go-to pizza. But pork no more, as I can only imagine every part of the pig from the tip of its snout to the skin around its anus is ground into sausage, hot dogs, bologna, etc.

I went to a chicken sausage demonstration at the Pizza Expo to see a cool rock star chef make some of what I thought was a healthier version of sausage. I was avoiding red meat at that point on my journey and wanted to enjoy sausage but by eating healthier chicken sausage.

Well, much to my dismay I saw the chef grind a lot of fat and skin into the sausage, he said it should be a minimum of 30%, in order to make the sausage moist and flavorful. I never ate chicken or turkey sausage again.

Feces on Meat

According to a petition to the USDA by the Physicians Committee for Responsible Medicine:

> *"Inconsistent with its statutory mandate, USDA regularly passes at inspection meat and poultry that is contaminated with feces. Although USDA implements a "zero tolerance" policy for fecal contamination, this policy applies to visible fecal contamination only. The result is that fecally contaminated meat and poultry products pass inspection as long as the feces on them are not "visible" to the naked eye.*
>
> *This inspection policy conveys a misleading promise of "wholesomeness." Feces may contain roundworms, hair worms, tape worms, and leftover bits of whatever the animal excreting the feces may have eaten, not to mention the usual fecal components of digestive juices and various chemicals that the animal was in the process of excreting. Americans deserve fair notice that food products deemed "wholesome" by USDA would be deemed disgusting by the average consumer and adulterated under any reasonable reading of federal law."*

The reality is that most animals raised for slaughter for

meat production have been living, eating, breathing and sleeping in a poop contaminated environment. You know this if you have ever been within a mile of a facility containing these animals you can barely take a breath the stench is so strong. I was recently driving through the panhandle of Texas and I had the vent closed but the stench was so strong it still infiltrated my car as I passed by a few hundred yards away.

So I am guessing these animals do not receive bubble baths in antibacterial soap before processing but instead are sent directly into plants where maybe they hose them down, maybe not. Then they are killed. Then their skins are torn off and they are gutted removing their organs and intestines which are full of poop.

So even if they are careful I would imagine some of the poop from the guts or from the coating of feces on the skin, gets onto the bare carcass which is then sent down the line for further disassembly. I have heard there is a "haze" hanging in the air in the facilities from all the fluids being drained from the animals and the activity that stirs it all up into the air as the animals are quickly cut up into pieces.

Then sharp objects like knives and saws undoubtedly slice the surface contamination into the flesh of the animal and onto and into whatever cuts of meat that will be eventually served onto plates somewhere.

I learned in food safety classes the reason that hamburger should be cooked thoroughly is because the surface contamination like E. coli are often ground into the meat. Whereas with a steak, the E. coli is still pretty much just on the surface of the meat so it can be served pink inside with less risk of the disease agent surviving the cooking process.

Consumer Reports, the independent not for profit organization, tested 300 packages containing 458 pounds of ground beef chosen at random from various stores and found:

> *"All 458 pounds of beef we examined contained bacteria that signified fecal contamination, which can cause blood or urinary tract infections. Almost 20 percent contained C. perfringens, a bacteria that causes almost 1 million cases of food poisoning annually. Ten percent of the samples had a strain of S. aureus bacteria that can produce a toxin that can make you sick. That toxin can't be destroyed—even with proper cooking.*

> *"Just 1 percent of our samples contained salmonella. That may not sound worrisome, but, says Rangan, "Extrapolate that to the billions of pounds of ground beef we eat every year, and that's a lot of burgers with the potential to make you sick." Indeed, salmonella causes an estimated 1.2 million illnesses and 450 deaths in the U.S. each year.*

> *"One of the most significant findings of our research is that beef from conventionally raised cows was more likely to have bacteria overall, as well as bacteria that are resistant to antibiotics, than beef from sustainably raised cows. We found a type of antibiotic-resistant S. aureus bacteria called MRSA (methicillin-resistant staphylococcus aureus), which kills about 11,000 people in the U.S. every year, on three conventional samples (and none on sustainable samples). And 18 percent of*

conventional beef samples were contaminated with superbugs—the dangerous bacteria that are resistant to
three or more classes of antibiotics."
https://www.consumerreports.org/cro/food/how-safe-is-
your-ground-beef

Somatic Cells (Pus) in
Dairy Products

Accepts to research by Dr. Michael Greger:

A ccording to research by Dr. Michael Greger:

"In the U.S. dairy herd, the dairy industry contin-ues to demand that American milk retain the highest al-lowable "somatic cell" concentration in the world. Somatic cell count, according to the industry's own National Mas-titis Council, "reflects the levels of infection and resultant inflammation in the mammary gland of dairy cows."

Just as normal human breast milk has somatic cells—most-ly non-inflammatory white blood cells and epithelial cells sloughed off from the mammary gland ducts—so does milk from healthy cows.

The problem is that many of our cows are not healthy. According to the USDA, 1 in 6 dairy cows in the United States suffers from clinical mastitis, which is responsible for 1 in 6 dairy cow deaths on U.S. dairy farms.

This level of disease is reflected in the concentration of somatic cells in the American milk supply. Somatic cell counts greater than a million per teaspoon are abnormal and "almost always" caused by mastitis. When a cow is infected, greater than 90% of the somatic cells in her milk are neutrophils, the inflammatory immune cells that form pus. The average somatic cell count in U.S. milk per spoonful is 1,120,000.

So how much pus is there in a glass of milk? Not much. A million cells per spoonful sounds like a lot, but pus is really concentrated. According to my calculations* based on USDA data released last month, the average cup of milk in the United States would not be expected to contain more than a single drop of pus.

As the dairy industry points out, the accumulation of pus is a natural part of an animal's defense system. So pus itself isn't a bad thing, we just may not want to have it in our mouth."

Almond and Cashew milk are probably sounding pretty good about now. There are nut based alternatives to most dairy products and most taste very good if not better.

Who Is Looking Out for Our Best Interests?

I really want to keep this book focused as much as possible on my selfish pursuit of the healthiest way to supply the one body I have in my life with substances that will keep me from suffering and hopefully live the longest life so I can enjoy my kids, grandchildren and maybe even great grandchildren.

And so I do not want to rant about government or industry or politics or greedy self-interests ... I want to as much as I can, Like Joe Friday on Dragnet used to say: "Just the Facts Ma'am."

But here are a couple glaring examples of government and industry allowing a misleading situation that most likely truly harms people. And one or both of these products are probably in the majority of kitchens in America.

Spray "Pam"® and Spray "I Can't Believe It's Not Butter"®. Both of which on their labels say they have Zero fat.

But in reality, the substances inside both packages are 100% Fat!

How can that be? Well it is from a combination of government labelling rules and ridiculously small serving sizes used on the labels by the manufacturers.

There is no way anyone who is using either of these products sprays them for "one third of a second". So the result is the consumer sprays what they need to coat the pan or coat the piece of toast in what amounts to many multiples of the suggested serving size and so they get fat in their food.

All the while they are deluding themselves they are having a fat free meal and then when they are huffing and puffing on the treadmill or laying sick and fat on the couch, are wondering why they can't seem to lose weight even though they think they are doing some of the right things.

And the government and the big processed food companies allow this to happen. So please use this example to realize that you need to take control of your own information stream and get down to the real science.

Because people with profit motives have huge incentives to manage the information you use in your decision making. They give you lots of messages helping you to rationalize and take a simple but unhealthy path.

Industry Created Confusion about Nutrition:
https://www.youtube.com/watch?v=J9vpohU4-zo&t=29s

How the Food Industry Works to try and Control Our Thoughts:

https://www.youtube.com/watch?v=KtdgjvO5qVM

Cheese Industry?:
https://www.youtube.com/watch?v=Opid_83-kSw

Why would bromate be added to flour? It is added to improve rise and elasticity of dough. In many countries around the world, bromate is a banned food additive. It is not banned in the United States. Why you ask?

In theory, because bromate is an oxidizing agent, it should be fully consumed in the bread baking process and there should be no bromate in the finished good.

However, if the conditions are off (think not baked long enough), some bromate will still be present in the baked good and that, in our opinion, is not good. You see, bromate has been linked to cancer in some lab studies and, while it is not a banned food additive, the FDA discourages its use by bakers.

USDA Conflicts:
https://nutritionfacts.org/video/dietary-guidelines-us-da-conflicts-of-interest/

Official Dietary Guidelines Advisory Committee Conflicts:
https://nutritionfacts.org/video/dietary-guidelines-advisory-committee-conflicts-of-interest/

And recent estimates put the average attention span of American's at between 8 and 12 seconds so it is unfortunate that most people will not take the time to look to see what the actual sources of information are for their nutritional choices.

The New Normal: Corner Drugstore

There is a large chain of drugstores that says they are "At the Corner of Happy and Healthy". However, when I walk in and look around, I think to myself the saying should be: "At the Corner of Processed and Reduced".

Most of the foods they will sell you are made up of processed ingredients where the carbs and fats have been separated from the fiber.

Then conveniently after someone may get a lifestyle disease, by consuming processed foods from the "drugstore", they can get the meds as prescribed by their doctor to treat the effects of the lifestyle disease at the same place!

Almost everything they sell is what Dr. Campbell refers to as "Reductionism" as all their products are processed and/ or reduced down into component parts. Which to me implies we think we are smarter than our amazingly complex bodies which obviously by the health issue statistics isn't going very well. Or, we are just looking for simple solutions: "silver bullets" to fix our issues.

The New Normal: Polyps are the New Black

Polyps are the New Black. "How many polyps did you have to have cut out during your colonoscopy?" seems normal now so I guess it is a normal subject at cocktail parties to compare how many polyps you've had cut out. Just like comparing cholesterol numbers etc. — the new normal.
https://www.mayoclinic.org/diseases-conditions/colon-polyps/symptoms-causes/syc-20352875

Should We All Get Colonoscopies at Age 50?
https://www.youtube.com/watch?v=4GDdWTnzVsU

Adventist Study of 96,000 Members in the U.S. and Canada Shows What Dietary Factors Can Reduce the Incidence of Polyps:
https://publichealth.llu.edu/adventist-health-studies/videos-and-media-reports/decrease-risk-colon-cancer

The New Normal: Joints Need to be Replaced

Joint replacement is also the New Black. "How is your new knee or hip working out these days?" seems normal now so I guess it is also a normal subject at cocktail parties—the new normal.

Why Our Joints Now Fail Sooner:
https://www.youtube.com/watch?v=WlK4eZQDxjg

Save Your Knees:
https://www.youtube.com/watch?v=7b9avQctpSk

Putrefaction: Rotting Dead Flesh Inside Us

Putrefaction of undigested animal protein in the colon can release hydrogen sulfide, the rotten egg gas associated with inflammatory bowel disease.

Typical meat eaters may get about 12 grams of undigested meat into their large intestine from each meal of meat which likely putrefies and creates hydrogen sulfide which is a poisonous gas.

The regular contact of this poison gas with the lining of the intestines is suspected to be one of the reasons that polyps form.

They used to think the small intestine digested all the meat but now research shows some is making it through to the large intestine where is putrefies. And then the gas most people expel smells like rotten eggs.

Bowel Wars:
https://www.youtube.com/watch?v=NUyi3UfzBYI

Resistant Starch and Colon Cancer:

https://www.youtube.com/watch?v=ZkrYeLy9xQM

Big Poops: Less Problems

Cultures that eat lots of fiber have almost no incidences of diverticulitis, hemorrhoids, colitis, irritable bowel syndrome, or Crohn's disease.

Consider the Scottish-born doctor who became the medical chief of Uganda and who wrote this best seller: *Don't Forget Fibre in Your Diet: To Help Avoid Many of Our Commonest Diseases. Denis Burkitt*. London: Martin Dunitz Ltd. 1979.

He saw that Africans who ate their traditional plant based high fiber diets had almost none of these diseases but once the same kind of people started eating like most of us do (western diet), the incidences skyrocketed.

Article from the British Medical Journal about fiber: https://www.ncbi.nlm.nih.gov/pmc/articles/PMC1796198/ pdf/brmedj02261-0052.pdf

Paleo Poo

The Paleo diet has some benefits like getting people off fast food, junk food and processed food. However, it is a hypothesis and doesn't really have any science to support what the proponents say cavepeople were consuming.
https://blogs.scientificamerican.com/guest-blog/human-ancestors-were-nearly-all-vegetarians/

https://www.smithsonianmag.com/smart-news/paleo-diet-may-need-a-rewrite-ancient-humans-feasted-wide-variety-plants-180961402/

And it really just seems like another "fad diet" where it seems to make sense and people still get to eat some of the foods they are in the habit of eating, like meats.

But some people kind of pick and choose from things they hear (I used to do the same thing!) like using coconut oil to cook while doing the "Paleo Diet". Well, any oil, including coconut oil, is a "processed food" meaning it was squeezed out and separated from the plant in which it grew.

If you put things in historical perspective, most processed

oils have only been around and commonly used for the last couple of centuries, and certainly were not available at the mini-mart down the street from the Paleo family's cave dwelling.

You can go into the science of the lauric acid in coconut oil or you can read the list of organizations that recommend not consuming it: Due to its high levels of saturated fat, the World Health Organization, the United States Department of Health and Human Services, United States Food and Drug Administration, American Heart Association, American Dietetic Association, British National Health Service, British Nutrition Foundation, and Dietitians of Canada advise that coconut oil consumption should be limited or avoided.

What We Can Learn from Fossilized Feces:
https://www.youtube.com/watch?v=4ZEZYu_7zR4&t=7s

Fossilized Poo:
https://www.youtube.com/watch?v=iVcSF5ecpmc

The Problem with the Paleo Diet Argument:
https://www.youtube.com/watch?v=wx0pOGVMnt-M&t=8s

What helped us to Evolve the Way we are:
https://sydney.edu.au/news-opinion/news/2015/08/10/starchy-carbs--not-a-paleo-diet--advanced-the-human-race.html

Paleo Diet Studies Show Benefits:
https://www.youtube.com/watch?v=KPt6ah__398&t=6s

Our Ancestors Ate Meat:
https://www.youtube.com/watch?v=x8o6q294vXU

EPIC Study:
https://www.youtube.com/watch?v=J0QIpp0nhXw

Dr. Klaper on the Paleo Diet:
https://www.youtube.com/watch?v=n663H-Acyp4

An Omnivore, a Paleo, and a Keto walk into a bar....

.......and overhear me explaining to an acquaintance how I lost weight after they asked me how it is that I look so much better.

The Paleo person tells me how much weight she has lost..... and how much she loves her Vitamix high-speed blender.....for her protein shakes....

The Keto person tells me how much weight she has lost but that she can only have one cocktail because that is all the "carbs" she is allowed...

The Omnivore tells me there is peer-reviewed science out there to support that humans are truly omnivores .... I said that was wonderful and I would love to read any study that shows an omnivore diet promotes longevity..... if she can show me where to find them....(haven't gotten anything yet).

They of course all asked me where I get my protein.....I told them the story about what gorillas consume......

But another joke came to mind when they walked away…..
you know the one where the wife asks the husband if her
dress makes her butt look big? And he says no that her butt
makes her butt look big!

All three of these women still looked like they were puffy
and inflamed. They may be losing some weight, but their
bodies didn't look like they were heading back towards
their natural shapes. They still had relatively big, thick,
squishy butts. Sorry kids, I calls 'em the ways I sees 'em…..

Are We Omnivores?

Some people are very convinced that we are Omnivores because we "can" eat animal products if we choose to, and trust me I used to choose to a lot. But the real question in my opinion should be: "Is being an Omnivore the best nutrition for longevity and pain free health?"

Yes, especially with the help of technology, we can eat a lot of different things without getting sick in the short term.

Knives and other tools allow for the effective dissection and separation of the "good" parts of the animals from the bacteria infested bowels. Refrigeration protects the "good" parts from bacteria growing to unsafe levels while the products are stored and transported, and then cooking techniques kill off any remaining remnants of bacteria that would cause issues with our digestive tracts.

I used to own a restaurant and the health department in their training and inspections pretty much treats raw animal products like hazardous materials because of the bacterial contamination.

Being able to eat many things probably helped some Paleolithic cave people to survive and not starve to death, but they were trying to survive and not worrying about longevity. (but archaeologists have found no fossils showing where they cooked with oil or had high speed blenders) https://www.youtube.com/watch?v=nS2_Q1NY8nU

Please Don't Call Me a Vegan

Choosing to eat a "vegan" diet and to call oneself a "vegan" is a choice, of course. But I now feel with what I have learned about the science of human nutrition and what I have experienced in my body as it reacts to different foods, that *I really have "no choice"* than to go with "plant based nutrition".

It only makes sense to me to consume food in a way that supports the biochemical and biomechanical processes in a way to give myself the best odds of feeling good and staying strong for as long as possible— hopefully free of pain and suffering all the way until the day I wake up dead!

So this is not a book about being a "Vegan." How I may "categorize" myself is a personal and private choice in my humble opinion, and I would prefer not to be "labeled" please. I've spent my whole life being labeled as a "redhead," with people making comments and cracking jokes. So maybe I'm a bit sensitive at this point. True as it may be, I am far more than a dietary label, as are you.

This is my story and I wanted to share it with you. All I ask is that you keep an open mind as I try to relate the science I have collected in a way that may connect with your awareness of how you are feeding your body and loved ones.

If the nutritional choices I have come to this far on my journey of digging into science must be categorized, the best terms I know and like so far would be "Nutrivore" or "Nutritarian".

Veganism, or the Vegan movement, lifestyle, or whatever you choose to call it, implies things not just about nutrition and how it relates to health, but also about animal welfare and the environment and ethical behavior.

And while I do not necessarily disagree with any of that, the primary purpose and focus of this writing is on finding credible science in the areas of biochemistry, biomechanics, biology, anthropology, population statistics and provable history of what we as humans ingest and how these various things affect our current and future health and promote longevity, hopefully with as little suffering and pain as possible.

So what being a *"Nutrivore" means to me is: "Seeking and applying the best scientifically derived evidence about human nutrition and how it affects vitality and longevity."*

Two years ago I made the decision to go fully with plant-based nutrition, and I couldn't love it more. I try to be as Whole Foods Plant Based(WFPB) as I can. But I still eat some processed foods and have had an occasional "Off Day" where I have eaten some food with animal products in them.

I am not perfect. But I have less and less urges to go off plant based as time goes on. I eat what I want to eat. I "can" eat anything I want, but I love feeling this way! And things like I used to eat just don't feel good on my palette anymore.

At some point very early on in the process of transitioning(a few weeks) it seemed like a switch was flipped and I just realized that I was feeling so much better all the time. And then, as I progressed, I could feel additional switches being flipped to the point now where I feel so darn good and do not want to go back.

What feels especially good is how people react when they see the new me. They say how good I look and that I must be working out or something. And I say: "Yes, or something."

Macho Consumption

Macho eating is one of the reasons men have, on average shorter lives than women. Dying young isn't macho, or necessary.

Why Women Live Longer... A Manly Diet:
https://www.youtube.com/watch?v=llMEv6aQgnw

In the United States 52% of men admit to experiencing Erectile Dysfunction (ED), but since it is embarrassing to talk about, the number is most likely much higher. Other sources say it is 40% by age 40 and 70% by age 70.

Let's learn about diet and manliness.

ED ... Cause and Cure:
https://www.youtube.com/watch?v=OVXzT_RBxFk

Masculinity and Meat:
https://www.youtube.com/watch?v=lKLFXQ0JO0o

It is an old term but "Canary in a Coal Mine" refers to when miners used to take a canary in a cage with them into the mines. When there was gas present, the canary would die before the men would start to pass out.

This would give them time to get out of the mine safely. In general, the dangerous gases in a coal mine are colorless and have no taste or smell. The methane gas that comes into your home has a smell because the gas company added it so you can sense the presence of natural gas.

ED is the "canary in a coal mine" when it comes to atherosclerosis, or the buildup of gunk, for lack of a better word, in your arteries. The artery to the penis is usually affected first because it is about half the size of the artery eventually affected in the heart.

Some cardiologists say that when you first experience erectile dysfunction you have about 10 years until the artery in your heart becomes clogged as well.

ED and Your Nuts:
https://www.youtube.com/watch?v=TewYl_Yl310

Foods to Improve Sexual Function:
https://www.youtube.com/watch?v=1kuL0TmYI9o

Female ED and Broken Orgasm:
https://www.youtube.com/watch?v=sv9U2ZBQYI0

Better at Sex?
https://www.youtube.com/watch?v=ZmW6bZxuS-TE&has_verified=1

Seems Like We Have been Conditioned to Ignore Potential Side Effects of Medicines:

I shake my head when I hear all the side effects on drug commercials.
https://www.salon.com/2016/03/14/drug_ads_2_part-ner/

https://www.psychologytoday.com/us/blog/meta-cognition-and-the-mind/201412/what-are-the-import-ant-side-effects-medication

https://www.wbur.org/commonhealth/2016/12/30/doc-tors-side-effects-medication
https://www.statnews.com/pharmalot/2016/10/14/side-ef-fects-medicines/

Here is a list of actual side effects I have garnered from the TV and internet ... the things they rattle off so fast on drug commercials and print in such small print on the screen that you can't read them:

- "Oily Anal Discharge."
- "An unusual urge to gamble or increased sexual urges and/or behaviors." "Visual, aural and tactile hallucinations."
- "Gas with oily spotting." "You may recognize it as something that looks like the oil on top of a pizza."
- "Loose stools" and "more frequent stools that may be hard to control."
- "Gynecomastia," the first four letters of which should make any man arch his eyebrow and feel wary. And with good cause, as gynecomastia means boobs. Boobs that can make milk.
- "Crying spells, rectal bleeding and bone fractures. Hepatitis, psychosis and hirsutism. Herpes."
- "Persistent, painful erection." "Ejaculation failure."
- It can kill your ability to handle sunlight. It's called "phototoxicity," which is characterized by rapid, second-degree sunburns.
- "Ruptured tendons." (We know someone whose Achilles tendon ruptured causing extreme pain).
- "...Hallucinations may occur..."
- "...Increased gambling, sexual, or other overpowering urges..."
- "Coma or death...And trouble swallowing."
- "Runny nose."
- "Dizziness."
- "Decrease in semen."
- "These changes may include gas with oily discharge, an increased number of bowel movements, an urgent need to have them, and an inability to control them."
- "Nasal sores, glaucoma, cataracts and nasal fungal

infection"
- "The way V********T works is not entirely understood."
- "...Benign but dangerous liver tumors. These benign liver tumors can rupture and cause fatal internal bleeding. In addition, some studies report an increased risk of developing liver cancer."
- "Asthma related death."
- "Nausea, sleep disturbance, constipation, flatulence, and vomiting."
- "suicide ideation."
- "Depressed mood, trouble concentrating, sleep problems, crying spells, aggression or agitation, changes in behavior, hallucinations, thoughts of suicide or hurting yourself."
- "Sudden numbness or weakness, especially on one side of the body."
- "Blurred vision, sudden and severe headache or pain behind your eyes, sometimes with vomiting."
- "Hearing problems, hearing loss, or ringing in your ears."
- "Seizure (convulsions)."
- "Severe pain in your upper stomach spreading to your back, nausea and vomiting, fast heart rate."
- "Loss of appetite, dark urine, clay-colored stools, jaundice (yellowing of the skin or eyes)."
- Severe diarrhea, rectal bleeding, black, bloody, or tarry stools.
- Fever, chills, body aches, flu symptoms, purple spots under your skin, easy bruising or bleeding.
- Joint stiffness, bone pain or fracture.
- "Sleep eating" — some having no memory of their

odd behavior upon waking. Yet as time passed (and the side effects continued to worsen), the FDA slapped this drug's medication guide: "After taking this drug, you may get up out of bed while not being fully awake and do an activity that you do not know you are doing. The next morning, you may not remember that you did anything during the night."

- "Depression, hostility, and suicidal thoughts."
- "Serious neuropsychiatric events, serious skin reactions, cardiovascular events, night terrors, insomnia, nervous system disorders, and eye disorders."
- "....Falling asleep while engaged in activities of daily living, including the operation of motor vehicles, which sometimes resulted in accidents."
- "....The drug caused permanent muscle and nerve damage."

I have to ask: How much do they pay people to be in the clinical trials for these potential drugs with all these crazy dangerous possibilities???

I think one of my favorite lines in all of that is: "...benign but dangerous." Huh? Really? The lawyer who wrote that should get a raise.

As opposed to the lists of side effects for substances used as medicines for health problems, there are no side effects for consuming only plant based unprocessed foods. Ok, well, maybe some gas during the transition as the microbiome adjusts to more fiber.

Medicine and Health are Different Things

A key difference between public health and medicine is that medicine emphasizes disease treatment and care, while public health emphasizes disease prevention and health promotion. However, the primary goal of medicine is to provide treatment and medical care for individuals who have already developed a disease.

https://study.com/academy/lesson/public-health-vs-medicine-differences-similarities.html

I know a nice older lady who lives near me who was trained as a nurse, and no doubt knows a lot about the application of medicine and medical techniques, which is called "health care." But in my observation, she also seems to have no clue about healthy eating habits or a healthy lifestyle.

She has been "sick" for years and is a living testimonial to the ability of the medical profession to keep someone alive and functioning with the application of drugs, surgeries and other techniques.

Too many people like to think everything can be solved by the magic of modern medicine. Just give me the right pills and they can go on eating whatever they want.

Or they blame health problems on genetics because "my dad or my grandpa had that same problem." Of course, he may have had that same problem because he probably ate the same crap and handed down the eating habits to the next generation.

Sometimes I pick up things from the grocery store for this nice lady and it just makes me crazy. She wants a gallon of hard to digest 2% dairy milk (because she thinks it is healthy) and the largest bottle available of an anti-diarrhea medication which she likely wouldn't need it if she stopped drinking milk all the time. Too many live in a vicious cycle like that.

Got Milk???.....Food Pyramid???:
https://www.youtube.com/watch?v=0O-ehIkwGME

Bone Fractures:
https://www.youtube.com/watch?v=4QIQGoGyNF0

Blue Zones Illustrate the Difference Between Health and Health Care:
https://www.youtube.com/watch?v=zTeYOLhkP9U

Whoa Nellie! - Flesh Eating Genital Infection?

The side effect that stopped me in my tracks was on a TV commercial for a personal injury lawyer trying to get clients who have been injured by a flesh eating genital infection from taking a particular medication. Seriously?

Certain diabetes drugs must warn of deadly flesh eating genital infection, FDA says. ... Necrotizing fasciitis is a rare bacterial infection commonly known as "flesh eating bacteria," according to the Centers for Disease Control and Prevention.

People actually take a medication where this is the possible side effect? But they are most likely resistant to trying to go with plant based nutrition for even a few weeks to see how they feel? And to see how it affects their blood sugar and insulin requirements?

To do something where the only side effect might be a little more gas (until your gut biome adjusts)? I don't understand people's choices.

I Need to Tell You that I
Have Cancer

I have cancer cells in my body—no doubt about it. My lifestyle, eating habits, and exposure to the sun, chemicals and environmental toxins, and the toxins that were bio-accumulated in the meat I consumed. And I used to smoke pot, cigarettes and the occasional cigar. So there is almost 100% statistical chance.

Cancer takes decades for the cells to mutate, multiply and grow, so I am certain I have some in there somewhere. I recently took a blood test where I paid extra to be tested for three cancer markers and two out of the three were elevated ... thankfully not Into the danger zone ... but still elevated.

So the question I have to ask myself is do I consume nutrition that has been shown to promote cancer cell growth thereby ignoring the science I have learned? Or do I consume nutrition that has been scientifically shown to fight cancer cell growth? Do I feed it or fight it?

I want my healthy cells and functions—my immune system—to win the fight.

I am now older than when my father died from cancer.
As a heavy smoker most of his life there was an obvious reason for his death, but he also let his general health go down. He sold his business, retired, and was no longer physically active.

He also started drinking more, and over the last 9 or 10 years of his life he got weak and overweight. His body no longer had the strength to fight off disease.

The temptation would be for me to say my fate is determined by genetics and that "life is short" so I should just enjoy myself. But what is enjoyable about getting sick just because I want to eat some different things? I want to feel the best I can for as long as I can.

But I was also exposed to dangerous substances—
I could have cancer or tumors lurking and growing inside me from the now banned chemicals that we sold at our family's store and wholesale company.

I used the chemicals that were mixed to make "agent orange" and occasionally had to clean up broken bottles of them and other nasty stuff. I breathed a lot of lead in the air from gasoline engine exhaust fumes and I washed my greasy hands in gasoline after helping my grandfather repair small engines.

I watched a story about Steve Jobs by Dr. McDougall who proposes that Steve's cancer probably started from exposure to chemicals used in the manufacturing of electronic parts, starting in his teens.

Cancer may be discovered all of a sudden, but it doesn't start out that way. It lurks, and grows, and eventually starts to fester. And if you stay strong and healthy your body can fight it or heal it or keep it at bay.

Win The War on Cancer:
https://nutritionfacts.org/video/how-to-win-the-war-on-cancer/

Why Did Steve Jobs Die:
https://www.youtube.com/watch?v=81xnvgOlHaY

I am now older than when my mother had a stroke. Playing the odds, I am choosing to try and stay strong and healthy. I am 62, but feel better than when I was 40 and overweight.

Turning Cancer On and Off:
https://www.youtube.com/watch?v=mguepud-BoYA&t=110s

Protein in Meat and Dairy Do What to Us?
https://www.youtube.com/watch?v=yfsT-qYeqGM

Muddy Waters and Cognitive Dissonance

I woke up one morning to a headline on my Google news feed that said: "The Case Against Carbohydrates Gets Stronger."

Well of course that is just the headline many people need to eat a pound of bacon and butter. And of course many of us will not even read the specifics in this article where instead of referring to carbs in general, it refers to refined carbs found in processed foods:

"Here's how this hypothesis goes: Consuming processed carbohydrates (especially refined grains, potato products and sugars), causes our bodies to produce more insulin.

Too much insulin, one of the most powerful hormones, forces our fat cells into calorie-storage overdrive. These rapidly growing fat cells then hoard too many calories, leaving too few for the rest of the body. So we get hungry, and if we persist in eating less, our metabolism slows down.

Our findings suggest that a more effective strategy to lose

weight over the long term is to focus on cutting processed carbohydrates, not calories."

Yes, yes, yes … processed anything is not what our bodies were engineered to deal with properly. There were no processed foods while humans were evolving into our current form.

Cavemen didn't own blenders, juicers, or food processors. Or buy bags of flour, sugar, salt or bottles of oils. They certainly weren't picking up coconuts off the ground and squeezing out the oil so they could fry potentially healthy sweet potatoes into saturated fat bombs.

Saturated Fat Studies - Set Up to Fail:
https://www.youtube.com/watch?v=2Ftoy6jqxm8

There are a lot of messages floating around out there to help people rationalize anything. I call them "Muddying the Waters" or that "Oily Film of Misinformation Floating on the Surface of the Sea of Knowledge."

Many of us seem to easily rationalize that our genetics alone are what determines diseases. Or that we are just unlucky and were dealt a bad hand from the deck of cards of life…then we say:"Supersize that please!"

Popular rationalizations:

- The body generates more cholesterol than is in one egg
- My dad was an alcoholic so I guess I am one, too
- My mom has high cholesterol so it is genetic

- I have cut down on eating "red meat" and eat mostly chicken and seafood and turkey so I am eating pretty healthy.
- I am eating only grass-fed organic beef.
- The chicken is free range and antibiotic free
- These eggs are from cage-free chickens.
- That muscular guy at the gym says we need lots of protein
- Protein is only found in meat
- I only eat high-quality protein which is found in meat
- I could never give up my eggs in the morning
- I love a good steak; I could never give that up
- I eat mostly seafood and take fish oil pills
- I only eat dairy from animals which doesn't hurt the animals
- I have lost weight with my Keto diet
- I have lost weight after I went Paleo

So what is Cognitive Dissonance?:
https://www.youtube.com/watch?v=yNerOJxtBh0

But the headlines can be irresponsible as they will help people to continue to justify continuing bad habits or even to start trying the very dangerous ketogenic diets that come in a number of names and forms.

(Author with an MD behind his name but no background in the science of nutrition says: "Potato Chips are OK!!! ....and by the way here is also a link where you can buy my book and buy supplements from me...")

So yes, when we slam our bodies with processed carbs, or oils, or proteins, our bodies are engineered by evolution to store anything extra somewhere in the form of fat, because people who managed to survive starvation in the winters or droughts had their genes passed on.

So Many Misconceptions and Myths about Nutrition:

L et's take Potassium. So many people think bananas should be eaten to get potassium. In reality, many other foods such as avocados and raisins have more potassium than bananas, so getting enough into your diet really isn't much of an issue if you eat fruits and vegetables.

But the marketing people for the banana industry should get a lifetime achievement award or something for planting this idea firmly in the minds of consumers.

98% of American Diets Deficient in Potassium:
https://www.youtube.com/watch?v=kVS2uoL74vQ

Potassium and Autoimmune Disease:
https://www.youtube.com/watch?v=kbwdsK7o0p4

Potassium to Reduce Stroke Risk:
https://www.youtube.com/watch?v=U3tY9f_AZ2s

Preventing Strokes:
https://www.youtube.com/watch?v=Fs4r9HmJXFs

Top Potassium Rich Foods:
https://www.youtube.com/watch?v=Fs4r9HmJXFs

Protein, Soy, Supplements and Other Myths:
https://www.youtube.com/watch?v=owhXsFvn-MC8&t=1154s

How the Food Industries want us to Not Think:
https://www.youtube.com/watch?v=J9vpohU4-zo

And the Dairy Industry Wants Us to Think Soy is Unhealthy:

I have been eating a lot of soy since I went plant based 2 years ago and my "Man Boobs" are actually getting smaller. My belly is getting smaller. I am getting smaller by being less round and more flat.
https://www.vice.com/en_us/article/vdb383/no-eating-soy-isnt-going-to-give-you-manboobs

So here are some links to actual non mythical science about soy:
https://www.hsph.harvard.edu/nutritionsource/soy/
https://www.drfuhrman.com/get-started/eat-to-live-blog/137/dont-fall-for-the-myths-about-soy
https://medium.com/impossible-foods/soy-facts-myths-and-why-its-in-our-new-recipe-12815b4997cf
https://www.todaysdietitian.com/newarchives/040114p52.shtml

We Need Dairy to Get
Our Calcium?

The first question is how did humans or their ancestors or our genetically similar cousins get calcium before we started milking and using cow's milk for human consumption about 10,000 years ago?

The second question is, why do populations with the highest levels of consumption of dairy also have the highest incidence of osteoporosis?

Dairy Consumption:
https://nutritionfacts.org/2017/01/31/why-is-milk-con-sumption-associated-with-more-bone-fractures/

Causes and Cures for Osteoporosis:
https://www.youtube.com/watch?v=0BR2bxQ7Hxc

9 Dairy Myth Perpetuations:
https://www.plantbasednews.org/opinion/world-milk-day-top-9-lies-the-dairy-industry-told-you

Are Dairy Free Diets Dangerous?:
https://www.youtube.com/watch?v=jyzYwVtvgEI

Got Milk? Let the Calves Drink It! (Pus and Manure in Milk) :
https://www.youtube.com/watch?v=x_CAqpBnd5E

Dissecting Industry Funded Misleading Studies:
https://nutritionfacts.org/video/how-the-dairy-industry-designs-misleading-studies/

Eggs are Wholesome and Healthy right?

According to communications with the egg industry marketing people uncovered using the Freedom of Information Act the United States Department of Agriculture says that not only can eggs not be called healthy they can't even be called safe. https://nutritionfacts.org/2015/03/26/peeks-behind-the-egg-industry-curtain/

Eggs are a huge source of saturated fat, cholesterol, and arachidonic acid which is highly inflammatory.

It Isn't Just About Cholesterol and Fat, It's About TMAO Too

So by the responses I get from a lot of people, I hear over and over that they think they are eating pretty good because they have cut down on red meat, or they say they don't eat much meat, or they say they only eat seafood and some chicken, or they make their chili with ground turkey now, or or or....I have heard a lot of similar responses.....

And I get it, I was in the same camp for years. I was doing pretty well, good numbers, not taking any medications, feeling pretty good. But even cutting down still means the gut is still being fed to produce a substance called TMAO and of course hydrogen sulfide gas which is the rotten egg smell that can clear a room.

The Surprising Link Between the Gut and Heart Health

S cience has long recognized that what we eat plays a critical role in our heart health. Now the details of this complex connection are coming into focus.

One of the more intriguing recent discoveries has to do with the role of the gut microbiome—the trillions of microbes that reside in the GI tract and influence health by helping digest food, making vitamins, and providing protection against disease-causing microorganisms.

Recently Cleveland Clinic researchers reported findings from several studies involving people and animals, that the gut microbiome directly changes the function of blood platelets, influencing the risk for heart attack and stroke.

Here's how it works: When people ingest certain nutrients, such as choline (abundant in red meat, egg yolks, and dairy products) and L-carnitine (found in red meat as well as some energy drinks and supplements), the gut bacteria that break them down produce a compound called trimethylamine (TMA). The liver then converts TMA into the compound, trimethylene N-oxide (TMAO).

The trouble with TMAO is that data show high levels contribute to a heightened risk for clot-related events such as heart attack and stroke—even after researchers take into account the presence of conventional risk factors and markers of inflammation that might skew the results.

In their most recent analysis, scientists showed that high blood levels of TMAO were associated with higher rates of premature death in a group of 2235 patients with stable coronary artery disease. Those found to have higher blood levels of TMAO had a four-fold greater risk of dying from any cause over the subsequent five years.

The implications are intriguing. Taken together, the new studies suggest that positively altering the gut microbiota may help to reduce damage to blood vessels, resulting in a stronger cardiovascular system, and they point to targets for potential new heart disease therapies.

The insights also underscore the potential power of TMAO testing, which can help patients determine if their gut microbiome is contributing to their risk for heart disease and whether they might benefit from limiting foods that contain the building blocks of TMAO. TMAO tests currently are only available through the Cleveland HeartLab.

To lower your TMAO levels, consider minimizing the consumption of full-fat dairy products, including whole milk, egg yolk, cream cheese, and butter; both processed and unprocessed red meat (beef, pork, lamb, and veal), as well as nutritional supplements and energy drinks containing choline, phosphatidylcholine (lecithin), and/or L-carnitine.

Vegetarians and vegans, who avoid meat products, for instance, produce little TMAO.

In general, consuming a diverse diet rich in plant foods and fiber may be helpful. When Cleveland Clinic researchers fed mice a diet rich in TMAO producing nutrients, they identified a compound called DMB capable of minimizing TMAO produced from their gut microbiota.

In fact, when DMB was added to their drinking water, they found TMAO levels and the formation of arterial plaques both declined. DMB may be found naturally in many Mediterranean diet foods, including red wine and extra virgin olive oil.

Such an eating pattern may turn out to be key to cultivating a healthy human gut microbiome—one that will fend off a number of potential illnesses, including heart disease, America's chief health threat.

I must say, I am feeling great, my numbers are great, and I am learning about the biochemistry. One of the key things that has convinced me to go all the way and eliminate all animal products is TMAO and how changing the flora in our gut biome is so important to changing what is flowing through our blood and how much it can affect our cardiovascular systems:

https://www.youtube.com/watch?v=dmMr8Foek-jk&t=102s
https://www.youtube.com/watch?v=A-kRUdspiSI&t=31s

Dangers of Eating Meat even Once a Week: https://www.

youtube.com/watch?v=kdJCP4j33pw

Seafood

I was a "Pescatarian" for a long time because I thought I was being healthy by consuming lots of seafood. I was doing pretty good and felt okay, but not amazingly great like I do now.

So fish oil and olive oil are supposedly "good oils" but let's face it they are still oils, processed foods, that our body was not engineered through evolution to safely process and use as fuel.

But seafood has other issues that I learned about when I took a deep dive into the science after one of our favorite customers died from ALS or Lou Gehrig's disease. This science on the issue really tells about bioaccumulation in the food chain.

Contributor to ALS: BMAA (Neurotoxin)
https://www.youtube.com/watch?v=SLVUfYEnVvs

More science and history about ALS and BMAA:
https://www.youtube.com/watch?v=9JzpotmloYE

More studies about BMAA:

https://www.youtube.com/watch?v=wcGr1WUCIf4

Mercury:
https://www.youtube.com/watch?v=M30cmiOomKg

False Teeth

My parents lost all their teeth and had false teeth, something that didn't seem to happen historically until the industrial revolution started refining foods, especially sugars.

I could have rationalized it was genetics and ignored the science that regular brushing and other types of oral care help prevent decay. It seems we are more willing to accept the science if we can actually see the results like with skin care or with oral care.

Dental Health:
https://www.youtube.com/watch?v=q8BKmlTLwUo
(Please note that Diet Coke® took first prize for softening tooth enamel.)

On the Fence

I get a lot of people responding to me saying: "But I don't eat that much meat. I have cut way down and I don't eat much red meat, mostly fish and chicken and turkey. That's good, right?"

I used to be that way and think that until I looked at the science.

Scary Truth about eating Chicken:
https://www.youtube.com/watch?v=rOLGG9Xr9fc

Salmonella in Chicken and Turkey:
https://www.youtube.com/watch?v=OiTs-A_IVjA

Superbugs in Chicken:
https://www.youtube.com/watch?v=RHfa4R3JChM

Chicken Salmonella Outbreaks:
https://www.youtube.com/watch?v=oOTZnwtt1DE

A lot of smokers thought and said similar things when the science came out about tobacco use. I'm sure they said things like oh I've cut down to half a pack or switched to filtered cigarettes or I only smoke when I go out, to be sociable.

Chronic Inflammation

Chronic inflammation is the "common denominator" of age-related diseases such as heart disease, many cancers, and Alzheimer's disease.

Inflammation of Aging:
https://www.youtube.com/watch?v=Dj_MaHa2NDY

Now you're probably familiar with inflammation on the surface of your body (sunburn) as local redness, heat, swelling and pain. But what you may not know is this: Inflammation also happens on the inside of your body, and this is where it can be the most dangerous to your health.

Inflammation is characterized by an increased blood flow to an area of infection or injury. In this process, your blood carries white blood cells, nourishment and repair cells to the injury site to aid in recovery. But when inflammation persists, it can actually damage your body and cause illnesses.

So what causes chronic inflammation? Stress, lack of exercise, genetic predisposition, and exposure to toxins are all common culprits. However, there's another major cause that's often overlooked: the foods that you put into your body.

Americans love pro-inflammatory foods ... the typical American diet is rich in animal protein, which is a source of arachidonic acid — a polyunsaturated omega-6 fat that can increase inflammation. Arachidonic acid generates a number of potent inflammatory compounds, including the following:

Prostaglandins
Prostacyclins
Leukotrienes
Thromboxanes

It's really important for people with inflammatory conditions to do everything they can to avoid increasing arachidonic acid levels.

Below is a short list of foods that anyone with an inflammatory condition should limit or even avoid entirely:

Red Meat – especially fatty red meat
White Meat – chicken, duck and wild fowl
Dairy – any animal milk
Eggs – avoid the yolk
Cheeses – especially hard cheeses
Certain fish – tilapia, catfish, yellowtail

Please note that a healthy diet usually contains a balance of omega-3 and omega-6 fatty acids. Omega-3 fatty acids help reduce inflammation, and some omega-6 fatty acids tend to promote inflammation.

Unfortunately, the typical American diet tends to contain far more omega-6 fatty acids than omega-3 fatty acids. Fixing this balance can go a long way toward easing inflammation.

What foods are anti-inflammatory? Fortunately, nature offers us plenty of foods that can help ease inflammation. Even better, these foods work without side effects while supplying us with essential vitamins and minerals that can boost our overall health:

Reducing Inflammation:
https://www.youtube.com/watch?v=rhdWlkGnKcw

Dr. Weil on Inflammation and Omega-3 Fatty Acids:
https://www.youtube.com/watch?v=RO_5vqMW4rU

Life is a Bowl of Cherries:
https://www.youtube.com/watch?v=pkPhH1RSkds

Purple Potatoes:
https://www.youtube.com/watch?v=dJm9VNdfJz8

What the Heck About Gluten

Only one in 133 people actually develop celiac disease. Less than 1%.

But about a 33-40% of people do have the genes that may cause them to have "sensitivity" to gluten.

One in three people have the genetics where they could progress to celiac, but there are many other factors that influence whether someone with the genetic predisposition actually progresses to have the disease.

Is Gluten Sensitivity Real?
https://www.youtube.com/watch?v=jQIkaPplCxY
How to Diagnose Gluten Intolerance
https://www.youtube.com/watch?v=kcSqCHZPB4k

Many people have self diagnosed based on some popular books.

Some people feel they have improved by giving up gluten but they don't have celiac and possibly aren't even sensitive to gluten. They are experiencing what is called an error of attribution.

This is Dr. Popper reviewing the research and putting it

into context:
https://www.youtube.com/watch?v=IsVv2FsgJic

Just for fun, let's also listen to Dr. Pam Popper, a well-known nutrition researcher talk at the beginning of this video, about having an intern help her to read and research all the sources cited by the author in the book "Wheat Belly":
https://www.youtube.com/watch?v=GBUnEFiU-w4s&t=563s

Or Dr. Neal Barnard another well regarded researcher talks about Grain Brain:
https://www.youtube.com/watch?v=21D8wtAHWJg

Categories of People who should Not Eat Wheat & Gluten
https://www.youtube.com/watch?v=c5fxa-O141g

Three Reasons Gluten Intolerance May Not be from Gluten
https://www.youtube.com/watch?v=n-x0Vbbjdo0

Gluten Free Diets
https://www.youtube.com/watch?v=qBXE28jMWdY

Our Mandy was Sick:

Our dog, Mandy was acting sick and was making some toxic messes in the house, which was out of character for her.

So we took her to the vet near our home where she has been getting her routine care for most of her life.

They immediately started talking about testing for cancer which would cost over $800 and chemotherapy that would cost thousands.

We loved Mandy, but were hesitant to spend that much money. We were also concerned the chemo would make her suffer.

But we are members of a barter organization, so we decided to see if they had any vets in the program for a second opinion.

This second vet turned out to be a great guy. Like an old country doctor, so to speak, even though he wasn't that old.

He said we could start out with some simpler and less expensive options and then maybe get to the tests and chemo that the other vet had mentioned if these options did not work.

He took some samples, gave her some pills and gave us some digestive relief food that had to be bought through a vet.

Things cleared up fairly quickly, and she went back to feeling better and to making nice little "doggie loggies", if you know what i mean.

That worked for about a year and a half before the toxic messes returned.

We took her back to the vet and she got some tests, tried some different food that she didn't like, took some pills that worked for a while and then the lightbulb went off over my head.

There are so many different breeds of dogs, with so many different genes how could a vet really know and keep track of how diet affects each breed? So I thought to call the rescue people for Mandy's breed which was Bichon Frise.

The woman I spoke to sounded like a sweet little old lady, and she loved talking about her Bichons; we talked for almost an hour. She said yes that Mandy's condition, which she said was likely a meat allergy, happens sometimes in older Bichons and suggested I try feeding her the following: canned pumpkin for food, and banana slices for treats, and sometimes feeding her green beans from a can.

She referred me to some websites and blogs devoted to the Bichon Frise breed where I could read more about their health and nutritional advice.

It worked like a charm. Mandy felt better again and her poops went back to nice little orange and sometimes green "doggie loggies".

She was that way for over a year and a half and was doing great! My little white curly haired waggy-tailed Vegan!

After a year or so she got tired of pumpkin and I looked on the internet on Bichon rescue websites and canned peas were suggested. Legumes, high in fiber and protein!

She loved them! (She also loved canned green beans and oatmeal and broccoli, and apple slices, etc.) Canned peas were her favorite and she was doing well for almost 2 more years to the age of 16 and a half until she woke up one morning and couldn't move and was clearly suffering. At that point we had her put down.

Study on Vegan Dogs:
https://v-dog.com/blogs/v-dog-blog/veterinarian-publish-es-study-on-vegan-dogs

The Other "White Meat":

The beef industry commissioned a review of randomized controlled trials on the effects of beef versus chicken and fish on cholesterol levels published over the last 60 years.

They found that the impact of beef consumption on the cholesterol profile of humans is similar to that of fish and/or poultry—meaning that switching from red meat to white meat likely wouldn't make any difference.
https://nutritionfacts.org/topics/beef/

I gave up the regular consumption of most red meat years ago thinking it was worse, so this explains why my total cholesterol number did not drop until I went with only plant based nutrition.
https://www.huffpost.com/entry/vegetarian-protein-complete-meat_n_5a90357ae4b01e9e56bb3224

How do we know that Cholesterol causes Heart Disease?:
https://www.youtube.com/watch?v=IUrP-g9TYdQ

Optimal Cholesterol Level:
https://www.youtube.com/watch?v=lakaozfALho

Nuts to YOU!!!!:
https://www.youtube.com/watch?v=5bmKEHVdbmY

U.S. Court of Appeals: False Claims about Eggs:
https://www.youtube.com/watch?v=8g8ASQZ0dZw

Getting to the Legitimate Scientifically Valid Information:

First off, it is important to recognize that scientific information is an evolving and often expanding subject. (Which unfortunately seems to allow many people to rationalize that science is coming up with "cures" so they don't need to modify their behavior.)

There are enormous profits to be made, so there are many who use old or sketchy science to develop and sell things claiming "science" to justify the use of these products. Or, there are enormous established industries that use "science" and "soundbites about science" to help people rationalize the use of their products.

Google is an efficient way to wade through lots of information, and YouTube (owned by Google) is a place where people have posted videos of researchers, scientists, doctors, etc. present their findings and sources and methodologies at conferences etc.

Usually the presenters have distilled their lengthy books and papers down to an hour or so in order to get their most important findings across to the audience in the time that has been allowed to them by the conference organizers.

My digging and reading has helped me to identify a core group of concerned people who are trying to get the word out about the actual science of nutrition. These are the primary people who have helped me so much on my personal journey:

Dr. Michael Greger

Many of you may be familiar with Sheldon on the sitcom: *The Big Bang Theory*. He is one of America's favorite "geeks" ... and it just so happens there is a Sheldon in real life in the field of nutrition science: Dr. Michael Greger. He runs a not for profit called: *Nutritionfacts.org.*

The Story of the Not for Profit: Nutritionfacts.org
https://www.youtube.com/watch?v=G9Z-gKAvzOY

Dr. Greger is the "geek's geek" when it comes to the science of nutrition, and he even kind of looks like Sheldon.

I have tried to find articles or people who can debunk his work and to show he is biased or not intellectually or ethically honest, but I have not found it yet.
https://www.mcgill.ca/oss/article/news/dr-michael-greger-what-do-we-make-him

Dr. T. Colin Campbell

This American biochemist specializes in the effect of nutrition on long-term health. He is the Jacob Gould Schurman Professor Emeritus of Nutritional Biochemistry at Cornell University.

Campbell joined MIT as a research associate, then worked for 10 years in the Virginia Tech Department of Biochemistry and Nutrition, before returning to Cornell in 1975 to join its Division of Nutritional Sciences.

Dr. Campbell is trying to get nutrition considered by medical professionals.

https://www.youtube.com/watch?v=tmWoWOM16uE

Dr. Caldwell Esselstyn

"Caldwell B. Esselstyn, Jr., received his B.A. from Yale University and his M.D. from Western Reserve University. In 1956, pulling the No. 6 oar as a member of the victorious United States rowing team, he was awarded a gold medal at the Olympic Games.

He was trained as a surgeon at the Cleveland Clinic and at St. George's Hospital in London. In 1968, as an Army surgeon in Vietnam, he was awarded the Bronze Star.

Dr. Esselstyn has been associated with the Cleveland Clinic since 1968. During that time, he has served as President of the Staff and as a member of the Board of Governors.

He chaired the Clinic's Breast Cancer Task Force and headed its Section of Thyroid and Parathyroid Surgery. He is a Fellow of the American College of Cardiology.

https://my.clevelandclinic.org/departments/wellness/integrative/disease-reversal

Dr. Esselstyn presently directs the cardiovascular prevention and reversal program at The Cleveland Clinic Wellness Institute:

https://www.youtube.com/watch?v=5P4pk-UffE0
https://www.youtube.com/watch?v=Xg5zcy20AAI

Here is a video interview with Samuel L. Jackson that references working with Dr. Esselstyn:
https://www.youtube.com/watch?v=tkkD2jZZntc&t=175s

Here is a short video that quickly covers the important points put forward by Dr. Esselstyn:
https://www.youtube.com/watch?v=G75Xu-x9zuY

Dr. Dean Ornish, M.D.

Dr. Ornish is the founder and president of the non-profit Preventive Medicine Research Institute and Clinical Professor of Medicine at the University of California, San Francisco.

Dr. Ornish received his M.D. from the Baylor College of Medicine, was a clinical fellow in medicine at Harvard Medical School, and completed an internship and residency in internal medicine at the Massachusetts General Hospital. He earned a B.A. in humanities summa cum laude from the University of Texas in Austin, where he gave the baccalaureate address.

Dr. Ornish was appointed by President Barack Obama to the White House Advisory Group on Prevention, Health Promotion, and Integrative and Public Health in 2010 and, previously, by President Clinton to the White House Commission on Complementary and Alternative Medicine Policy in 2000.

He chaired the Google Health Advisory Council 2007-

2009.He has received numerous national and professional awards including being honored by *LIFE* magazine as "one of the fifty most influential members of his generation," being recognized as "one of the most interesting people of 1996" by *People*; and having been described in Forbes magazine as "one of the seven most powerful teachers in the world."

The Ornish diet, a critical component of the Ornish Program, was rated #1 for heart health by *U.S. News & World Report* in 2011, 2012, 2013 and 2014.
https://www.ornish.com/proven-program/the-research/

Nathan Pritikin

Nathan Pritikin attended the University of Chicago from 1933 to 1935, dropping out because of the depression. He became an inventor and a millionaire developing patents for companies such as Honeywell, General Electric and Bendix.

After being diagnosed with heart disease in 1955, he began searching for a treatment. Based on studies indicating that people in primitive cultures with primarily vegetarian lifestyles had little history of heart disease and western cancers, and medical data available during World War II detailing rates of disease in various countries he created a low-fat diet that was high in unrefined carbohydrates like vegetables, fruits, beans, and whole grains, along with a moderate aerobic exercise regimen.

His dietary and exercise regimen is called the "Pritikin Diet".

https://www.drmcdougall.com/misc/2013nl/feb/pritikin.htm

Brenda Davis R.D.
Brenda is a Canadian registered Dietician and is very passionate about promoting public health issues by way of education. Her website is a treasure of information including many recipes for each meal and snack of the day.
http://www.brendadavisrd.com/about-me/

Dr. Milton Mills
Dr. Mills is a Stanford Medical educated physician who is very passionate about public health. In my opinion he does the best job of presenting how the physiology of a carnivore is different form herbivores.
https://www.youtube.com/watch?v=nS2_Q1NY8nU

Dr. Pam Popper
Dr. Popper is a straight-talking professional who is not afraid to criticize national health organizations, government agencies, medical professionals, pharmaceutical companies, agricultural organizations and manufacturing companies, many of whom have agendas and priorities that interfere with distributing truthful information and promoting public health.
https://drpampopper.com/about-pam/

Dr. Kim Williams
Dr. Williams graduated from the University of Chicago in 1975 and the Pritzker School of Medicine at the University of Chicago in 1979. He has board certifications in internal medicine, cardiovascular diseases, nuclear medicine, nu-

clear cardiology, and cardiovascular computed tomography.[2] He has served on the faculty of the Pritzker School of Medicine, the Wayne State University School of Medicine in Detroit, Michigan, and since 2013 at Rush University Medical Center in Chicago, where he is the head of the cardiology department. He is a Fellow of the American College of Cardiology and served as its president from 2015 to 2016.
https://well.blogs.nytimes.com/2014/08/06/advice-from-a-vegan-cardiologist

Ray Cronise
Former NASA Scientist and Nutritional Science Geek
https://about.me/raycronise

Dr. Michael Klaper
Dr. Klaper is currently working to promote the study of nutrition in medical schools: https://www.youtube.com/watch?v=rzqimKcdLms

In 1987 Klaper appeared on the game show Jeopardy and won $11,000.
Really what else do you need to know?
https://www.doctorklaper.com/

Dr. Neil Barnard
Dr. Barnard received his medical training at George Washington University School of Medicine in psychiatry, where he began to explore vegan diets.

He is board certified by the American Board of Psychiatry and Neurology, a fellow of the American College of Cardiology and a lifetime member of the American Medical Association.

Barnard founded the Physicians Committee for Responsible Medicine (PCRM) in 1985 because he "wanted to promote preventative medicine."
https://www.pcrm.org/clinical-research

Dr. John McDougall
Dr. McDougall is a physician and nutrition expert who has been studying, writing, and speaking out about the effects of nutrition on disease for over 50 years. Dr. McDougall believes that people should look and feel great for a lifetime. Unfortunately, many people unknowingly compromise their health through poor dietary habits.
https://www.drmcdougall.com/

Dr. Alan Goldhamer, D.C.
Dr. Goldhamer is the founder and education director of TrueNorth Health Center in Santa Rosa, California. Under his guidance, the center has supervised fasts for thousands of patients and grown into one of the premier training facilities for doctors wishing to gain certification in the supervision of therapeutic fasting.
https://www.youtube.com/watch?v=TAtqz24_UeE

Mic the Vegan
Here is young vegan who is energetic, passionate, talks very fast and tries to be funny. Sometimes he is successful. But his real value is that he presents a lot of information in a short period of time and provides many links to the actual science he is presenting.

https://micthevegan.com/

I'm sure there are many more who are serious about provable science and are dedicated to getting the information out in order to advance public health, but the ones I have listed have helped me the most on my journey and I sincerely thank them and feel grateful for their work and dedication.

Sad Case: We Learned so much from the Okinawans, but now:

Okinawa was one of the Five Blue Zones identified by the researchers from the National Geographic project, but now they are suffering the ill effects of one of the USA's biggest exports: Fast Food.

According to Dr. Greger, fast food restaurants in Okinawa have contributed to the population going from being the thinnest sub-population in Japan to being one of the most obese. There are efforts in Okinawa to try and get the people to go back to eating the way they did in the past.

The Okinawa Diet:
https://www.youtube.com/watch?v=mryzkO5QWWY

Turning Apples into Sugar Water.....

Apples are very nutritious. We've all heard "An apple a day keeps the doctor away" and there science demonstrates it can be true. The most nutritious part of the apple is the peel, but every day millions of beautifully nutritiously compete apples are pressed and squeezed to make apple juice. While it may be a kid favorite, and something that moms think is better than soda, in reality it's not much better.

Apples are a good example of something that is very healthy when consumed as a whole food, where the sugars and nutrients are still attached to the fiber where they grew on the plant.

But when refined by squeezing into juice, they go way up to the top of the glycemic scale, where the fiber has been removed, most of the other nutrients have been removed, and what is left is basically flavored sugar water.

It races into a person's system and is not digested naturally and slowly where all the biochemical and biomechanical benefits of the whole food are available for use by the body to feed the cells properly and to aid in the "flow" of the digestive process.

Apple Peels Put to the Test:
https://www.youtube.com/watch?v=rkhlPYABYK8

History of our Ancestors, and Food

I've mentioned how closely we're related to gorillas elsewhere. Let's just start at about 4,000,000 years ago with our first ancestors that walked on two legs. Australopithecus were our first bipedal ancestors and transitioned us from the apes.

From fossils discovered and analyzed the face and dental anatomy suggests that australopiths were adapted for eating tough, hard-to-process foods such as tubers, nuts, seeds or roots. Their teeth look pretty similar to ours. https://www.nature.com/scitable/knowledge/library/australopithecus-and-kin-145077614

About 800,000 years ago, fossil evidence shows a dramatic increase in the size of the human brain due to genetic change in salivary amylase genes, which created enzymes allowing our digestive system to increase the amount of available glucose that feeds the brain.

The cooking of starchy foods also seems to have increased the bioavailability of glucose around the same time. https://sydney.edu.au/news-opinion/news/2015/08/10/

starchy-carbs--not-a-paleo-diet--advanced-the-human-race.html

The brain runs on pure glucose by the way, which really calls into question the low carb diets.

For *Homo sapiens*, the most robust statistical examination to date of our species' genetic links to "mitochondrial Eve" — the maternal ancestor of all living humans—confirms that she lived about 200,000 years ago in Africa.

The study was based on a side-by-side comparison of 10 human genetic models that each aim to determine when Eve lived using a very different set of assumptions about the way humans migrated, expanded and spread across Earth. The oldest modern human remains are two skulls found in Ethiopia that date to this period.

At about 150,000 years ago, humans were possibly capable of speech. 100,000-year-old shell jewelry suggests that that people developed complex speech and symbolism.

About 12,000 years ago, modern humans reached the Americas.

Then 10,000 years ago, agriculture developed and spread. The first villages were established, and possibly the domestication of dogs.

About the same time, the first evidence of dairy consumption was found. But more widespread consumption didn't happen until a couple of thousand years later.

The genetic adaptation that enabled some early Europeans to drink milk without getting sick has been mapped to dairying farmers who lived around 7,500 years ago in a region between the central Balkans and central Europe. It was not a universal change. My sister still gets sick if she eats dairy as do about 67% of people on earth. 75% of African Americans are lactose intolerant.

The extraction of sugar cane juice from the sugarcane plant, and the subsequent domestication of the plant in tropical Southeast Asia sometime around 8,000 B.C.

The invention of manufacture of cane sugar granules from sugarcane juice in India occurred a little over two thousand years ago, followed by improvements in refining the crystal granules in India in the early centuries A.D. Then the spread of cultivation and manufacture of cane sugar progressed to the medieval Islamic world together with some improvements of production methods.

The spread of cultivation and manufacture of cane sugar to the West Indies and tropical parts of the Americas began in the 16th century, followed by more intensive improvements in production in the 17th through 19th centuries in that part of the world. The development of beet sugar, high fructose corn syrup and other sweeteners came in the 19th and 20th centuries.

Olives were first turned into olive oil about 8000 years ago and as early as 3000 BC in Mesopotamia, cooked meats and fish were preserved in sesame oil, and dried, salted meat and fish were part of the Sumerian diet.

The current expeller process for refining oilseeds into cooking oils was invented in Holland in the 1600s.

The earliest archaeological evidence for wheat seeds crushed between simple millstones to make flour dates to 6000 BC. The Romans were the first to grind seeds on cone mills.

In 1879, at the beginning of the Industrial Era, the first steam mill was erected in London. In the 1930s, some flour began to be enriched with iron, niacin, thiamine and riboflavin. In the 1940s, mills started to enrich flour. Folic acid was added to the list in the 1990s.

So for 99.75% of our walking on two legs ancestral existence, our predecessors did not consume dairy or processed foods such as carbs squeezed or milled away from the fiber, or oils extracted from plants.

In my mind this explains why our bodies are malfunctioning after consuming food this way. We are engineered to chew and digest the food to break it down and our bodies then use all the complexities of the food to feed our cells.

Pre broken down substances race into our systems, do not provide complete nutrition and cause havoc. And many of the nutrients that are in whole foods are stripped away from the processed end results.

I Don't Blame People for Not Knowing

The checkout lady at the grocery store asked me: "What are Smart Dogs®? I told her they are hot dogs flavored with the same spice as regular hot dogs but that are not made from ground up dead animals that were raised confined and sick from living in their own filth.

I say this not from my concern for animal welfare, but about the cleanliness and sense of what I put in my mouth. I don't want something that was living, eating, breathing, sleeping, drinking in a filthy smelly bacteria infested environment. Too many animals have to be treated with antibiotics to keep them from getting sick before they are disassembled using cutting tools that are covered in feces and bowel bacteria.

Even Kosher hot dogs, which are supposedly made from only the good parts of cattle, are still made from ground and heavily seasoned dead animals, then seasoned with salts and flavorful plant based substances.

Think about it, try to wrap your head around this: Things that season our meats are from plants, so things that were not raised in their own filth can be prepared with the same seasonings. I season TVP, seitan, tofu, tempeh, mushrooms, eggplant and other foods with many of the same seasonings that are used to make otherwise bland tasting meat taste better.

These foods may have had their roots in manure, but they weren't living down in it and it wasn't in the air and on the cutting tools when these plant based foods were cut up.

There are foods I get to eat again, now that I have a plant based diet, that I had stopped eating. Comfort foods like I grew up with: hot dogs, hamburgers, sloppy joes, meat tacos, chili, gyros, ham sandwiches, breakfast sausage, Italian sausage, beef brisket, etc.

I had stopped eating them when I started thinking about how and from what they were made. I can only imagine the "floor sweepings" and fatty grisly trimmings they push into the grinder that makes the hot dogs and sausages and other ground meats. Once I visualized that I became honest with myself and realized it was ... unacceptable for consumption.

Paul McCartney is of course famous for other things too, but for saying: "If slaughterhouses had glass walls then most of us would be vegetarian."

Have you ever been near a facility where they are raising animals for meat? You can barely breathe from the stench. So I decided I do not want to eat something that is raised in a filthy environment. Every breath that animal takes in is that horrible smelly air which must somehow permeate into the flesh of the animal that we are eating. Yuck!

Most animal foods are not eaten in their natural state, because in their natural state they are slimy and gross. Many people will not eat oysters because they are slimy and not attractive to look at.   But the stuff that is ground up and disappears into hot dogs and other prepared foods are also slimy, and nasty looking before they are seasoned and cooked, or mixed into things.

Even a boneless skinless chicken breast is slimy and kind of gross. Cooking a chicken breast without any plant based seasoning leaves it very bland and flavorless.

A few years back I was at the Pizza Expo in Las Vegas, and a "celebrity" chef was giving an hour long demonstration workshop on making Chicken Sausage. I was on my journey to eat healthier so I was interested in learning to make what I thought would be "healthy" sausage.

Well, I was very surprised to see him grind in some of the skin and fat and to say it was required if a juicy flavorful tender sausage was desired. He said that the sausage should be about 30% fat and skin for the best results.

When I looked at the actual numbers for chicken and turkey sausage or ground meat they really were not appreciably better than ground up pork or beef, still containing lots of saturated fat and cholesterol.
https://www.youtube.com/watch?v=RjNcvDxCvFk

I Was in the Moderation Camp
for a Long Time

When I think back to my "pescatarian, ovo, lacto" days (pre fully plant based), I can see how much fat I was consuming in the form of milk, butter, eggs, and cheese. So much cheese, I was a cheese-aholic!!

Cheese is addictive because the dairy proteins inside can act as mild opiates. Fragments of cheese protein, called casomorphins, attach to the same brain receptors as heroin and other narcotics.
https://www.drcarney.com/blog/entry/opiate-like-chemicals-in-cheese-are-physically-addictive
https://nutritionfacts.org/topics/cheese/

Moderation:
https://www.youtube.com/watch?v=X4oAqMpJ52I

I was putting the olive oil, avocado and cheese onto a lot of processed flour based bread and because olive oil is part of the Mediterranean diet I thought it was good for me and I was eating a lot of those cholesterol, saturated fat, choline and "arachidonic acid bombs" called eggs. Again, I thought I was eating well for my health. "All things in moderation," which was an okay place to start, but still bad.

Arachidonic Acid:
https://nutritionfacts.org/video/inflammatory-re-marks-about-arachidonic-acid/

Proof in my Pudding (or from losing my Pudding)

The "Proof is in the Pudding" has long been the phrase I think of when trying to determine if something is true or not. You can try to tell me why the pudding should taste good, but the proof is when I can taste the goodness for myself.

So I have actual real life statistical proof to relate what actually is working (cholesterol = 166) versus what someone tells you should work. And I hope to guide you to actual statistical evidence gathered from groups of thousands of real populations of people that helped me realize what I needed to do to be on this good path. By losing a lot of my "pudding" I have made significant progress toward my goal.

Here is a study testing a plant-based diet in a group of 64 women. It's similar to what I have been doing myself for the last two years. At the start of the study, all of the women were moderately or severely overweight. Participants

followed two simple rules: They set aside all animal products and kept oils to a minimum. They lost about a pound per week, without calorie counting or exercise. After two years, they maintained the weight loss.
https://www.pcrm.org/health-topics/weight-loss

MicroBiome Rebuilding:

On the typical American diet, with the consumption of meat and eggs and such, the colonies of bugs deep inside our digestive tracts produce a couple of nasty substances, hydrogen sulfide gas and TMAO.

I don't know when it exactly happened over the last two years, but I feel my gut microbiome has changed and the most readily evident thing that I notice is that I don't seem to be producing hydrogen sulfide gas any longer which has that characteristic sulfurous rotten egg smell to it.

In fact when I pass gas or eliminate in the morning there is hardly any smell to it at all. This is a significant change because back in the day I could clear a room. And unfortunately it lasted an incredible amount of time.

The bugs deep inside us:
https://getpocket.com/explore/item/how-the-western-diet-has-derailed-our-evolution-1101393416

How to Get Healthy Gut Flora and Avoid Inflammation:
https://www.youtube.com/watch?v=bQuElNkKJP4

TMAO and Changing the Flora in our Guts:
https://www.youtube.com/watch?v=dmMr8Foekjk&t=78s
https://www.youtube.com/watch?v=A-kRUdspiSI
https://www.youtube.com/watch?v=x3yp0oTd1Y-
A&t=173s

Playing the Odds:

So if I choose modern medicine to fight diseases, my use of these prescribed substances could cause not so pleasant to dangerous, to even life threatening side effects.

But if I use nutrition and exercise to prevent the diseases from progressing the potential side effects are possibly some extra gas. (Which I did have a bit of in the beginning, but it has gone away).

Microbiome:
https://www.youtube.com/watch?v=2ObAE52uMDU

Those Sensible Canadians:

Recently the Canadian Government came out with a fairly radical new "Food Guide" that is based more on science than ever before. How did they do it? Well, the panel assembled to create the new food guide was made up of scientists who were all independent of the food processing and agriculture industries.
https://www.bluezones.com/2019/01/news-canadas-new-food-guide-features-plant-slant-recommendations/

"Health Canada has grown a backbone and distanced itself from industry by excising some dubious advice that was clearly designed to mollify industry, such as the recommendation to drink two glasses of milk a day and consume at least two tablespoons of canola oil every day."
ANDRÉ PICARD , Globe and Mail

https://food-guide.canada.ca/en/

Reaction to Canada's Food Guide:
https://www.youtube.com/watch?v=lp4zWaLE_ik

The Path I've been on the last 24+ Months

When I decided to really try a completely plant-based diet, the first person I contacted was my favorite nephew Mickey. He gave me some tips on how to go plant based, as he had done it a couple of times before. One of his tips that has served me well is: "Don't be too hard on yourself; you will have some "off days" ... no big deal, just get back on it." He was right, and over time the off days have become less and less because I have just lost my desire for a lot of that stuff.

Now don't be thinking this took a lot of discipline. I'm not very disciplined at all. The first few weeks, I was already starting to feel better. And that's what kept me going. My skin cleared up (my nose was always breaking out) and I was dropping pounds. I was eating food that I really enjoyed and was pretty easy to prepare. (So seriously, if I can do it I think pretty much anyone has a chance.) There are recipes in the back of this book to get you started.

I really like what I am eating and I enjoy feeling so good, which makes it easy now.

After a few months on this path I was feeling better and better. As I lost more weight people were starting to say, "Wow you look so good." At that point I got a blood test and my total cholesterol was down to 170.

I had lost about 10 pounds without counting calories, without starving myself and I was never hungry. I was full and all the time I was eating delicious food and discovering more wonderful recipes so it just made me want to keep going and learning more and more about it.

Penn Jillette the magician tells what I want to tell you: https://www.youtube.com/watch?v=NelIXCuuSZ0

Once I got my mind into the actual science of nutrition then I started to understand how what we absorb affects how our bodies function. From then on it has been pretty easy for me to realize this made sense and I certainly was feeling better and losing weight so I wanted to keep following it.

Motivation to Keep on
This Path

I've credited him before, but a lot of my early motivation to keep doing it came from scientific information presented by Mic the Vegan (Mike) who is a passionate and humorous Vlogger on YouTube. Mike's videos helped me get past all the pseudo-science floating around out there—the kind mostly presented by "popular media" outlets. Here are some of my favorite videos by Mic that helped motivate me. I hope you'll find them helpful too.

Ten Amazing Body Transformations:
https://www.youtube.com/watch?v=APkUh7-JUpo

How Your Body Transforms on Plant Based Nutrition
https://www.youtube.com/watch?v=yKp8-X1zZqo

More Ways Your Body Transforms
https://www.youtube.com/watch?v=HAaK--L9tDk

Mic's How To Transition Guide
https://www.youtube.com/watch?v=Wofs3rFnggs

My Skin has Cleared Up a Lot!

Causes of Acne
https://www.youtube.com/watch?v=jd4BQu0-5FE&t=47s

So If You are Still Obsessed With Protein Sources:
https://greatist.com/health/complete-vegetarian-pro-
teins#1

Admittedly, I have crossed from being "Passionate" about
the biochemistry of nutrition to being "Obsessed"—just
ask any of my friends! But I'm serious about trying to help
you live a longer healthier life. And that's worth being passionate ... or even obsessive about.

Resistance and Getting to the "Tipping Point"

If you decide to join me on this journey towards healthier nutrition, I must warn you: people will think you are crazy. They think it is so foreign to what they know that they won't even consider it and think you shouldn't either. Or they think as I did, that they are already eating pretty well by giving up red meat or fast food and processed foods. Those are good steps for sure.

In the beginning—and maybe like you too—everything in moderation was my mantra. But then I realized moderation is like cutting down from a pack of cigarettes a day to half a pack. That didn't help my mom in the end, and it won't give you the full benefits either.

So my challenge in this book is to try to craft analogies and stories and explanations and present information and links for you to go to the actual science and hopefully be motivated to give "it" 3 to 4 weeks. And then you can make a decision based on whether or not you're feeling better.

I think if you really give it a valid try over 3 to 4 weeks

there is a pretty good chance you'll reach what I call the "tipping point" where you will notice some changes, some positive results, like losing some pounds, seeing your belly getting flatter, or your skin clearing up, or not having aching joints, and then you won't need me for motivation— you'll be on your way.

I think when I hit the 100 days when I had been through a whole cycle of cell regeneration, things really started to improve. I was sure it couldn't last because I felt so fantastic. But it did. And I want you to experience it too.

Confessions of a Doughnut Shop Owner:

Oh my, you should see what I have seen.

Doughnuts or donuts, are not food, they are wallpaper paste formed into circles, then fried in Trans Fats, then coated in various refined sugary flavored liquids which then all harden just enough to be shelf stable but quickly return to a paste form in your mouth when chewed and mixed with saliva.

I've made them, all kinds, at all hours of the night, for many hours on end, and I've seen too much. I will never eat one again. No one should.

Confessions of a Restaurant Owner:

Oh my, you should see what I have seen.

Ask any plumber who has had to work to open up a clogged kitchen drain at a restaurant about the type of material causing the obstruction. Most likely he will tell you it is hardened thick grease.

Most restaurants and commercial kitchens of all types are required to install grease interceptors to catch this nasty stuff so it does not make it into the municipal sanitary sewer systems where it can clog and cause havoc.

But as someone who has owned a restaurant for over a decade and has paid and watched plumbers do their work to reopen drains that, even with the interceptors, are clogged by the grease particles that are still suspended in the flow of liquids headed to the sewers, I can tell you it is nasty stuff, and that it resembles nothing I have purchased for the operation of my kitchen.

Huh? Then from where does it come? Well it is saturated fat which cooks out of the flesh, connective tissue, body fat, skin and bones of the animal products (a.k.a. meat) purchased for the preparation of the dishes we served.

And not all of it cooks out of the meat that makes onto the plates of the consumers. It is eaten and chewed and digested and absorbed and makes it into the blood of the human carnivores.

Stop Already! Ok! Ok!....
We Get Your Point.....

But how difficult is it to switch to this horribly restrictive "diet"???

- I don't consider it to be restrictive at all, I consume and have available for my pleasure a wide and expanding selection of cuisines and foods.
- What we consume are habits. It is changing some consumption habits from unhealthy piles of things to healthy piles of things.
- I consider it to be a fun and mind expanding adventure to learn about and find and make new things. Life is a journey grasshopper! Enjoy it and have fun with it!
- Payoff comes quickly. I wanted and still want to do it more and more.
- It isn't a "diet", they are not sustainable. It is a change in "lifestyle" habits so you do not get painful "lifestyle diseases".

Stop Going to the Gym Everyday

I try to go to the gym every day, and I try to work out. But mostly I go for my "Executive Workout" which is the steam room, the hot whirlpool, and then the dry sauna (because I like the wood smell) and then a nice shower, and boy do I feel great after.

But I walk past the same people everyday huffing and puffing on the treadmills and other machines, and I've seen the same people for years that still do not look healthy and still have big bellies or saddlebags etc.

My advice is they should take a day off and cook some healthy foods to have prepped to grab from your fridge. Veggie chili, or asian foods such as curries and dahls are tasty and very satisfying and very easy to make.

It is the 80/20 rule…...80% nutrition and 20% working out. I know your personal trainer may not like to hear that, but I've had discussions with people who have been long time fitness instructors. They admit that even dedicated exercisers sabotage their health by what they eat, even though they religiously go to spin classes etc.

So cook one day and get off the processed foods and the animal products. Just try it for three weeks and see how you feel. I lost seven pounds in the first three weeks and my face cleared up and I started to feel much better, even though I thought I was eating well before. Try it, no side effects!!!!

Abs Start in the Kitchen:
https://www.youtube.com/watch?v=cFoILYduzLI

Which Kills Cancer Cells Better, Diet or Exercise?
https://www.youtube.com/watch?v=pEQ8orjYNPA

Days Off, Every Once in a While

Some of you know I used to own a place that has really good thin crust pizza, which of course is one of my favorite things ever. The cheeses they use on that pizza are just great, so if I was working and the chef put out pizzas for staff dinner, well, I had to have some.

Most off days have been back to pizza or pescatarian. However, I've not been tempted to eat seafood since researching and learning about the link between consumption of seafood and ALS (Lou Gehrig's disease).

Eating Meat Once in a While:
https://www.youtube.com/watch?v=kdJCP4j33pw

Taste and Spit

If I have to taste something I will put it in my mouth and chew it a while and then spit it into a napkin. I use this technique at food shows for my work where I want to taste something but not put it into my digestive tract—some pleasure without adding to long term pain.

A minute on the lips, but it never gets to the hips!

Heart Attack Proof

My goal is to get my cholesterol down to 150 (or lower) which is said to be "heart attack proof.

Rather than hit the gym, I try to stay very active, ride my bicycle as much as I can, but for fun, not to exercise. But the 80/20 rule applies anyway. Health appears to be 80% nutrition and 20% fitnes. Now that I am feeling better I find myself motivated to try and do more fitness activities: walking, weights, etc.

Athletic Performance:
https://www.youtube.com/watch?v=fGwTD2cQzVY

Heart Attack Proof:
https://www.youtube.com/watch?v=N6nf9weAp0k

I really like Tomatoes:
https://www.youtube.com/watch?v=_hAtPXHJ5mY

The Kind of Success Story I Hear from Independent Sources:
https://www.everydayhealth.com/columns/my-health-

story/my-vegan-heart-how-changing-my-diet-changed-
my-life/

Aging Accelerated by Inflammation

What can we eat to reduce the chronic inflammation that accelerates aging?
https://www.youtube.com/watch?v=Dj_MaHa2NDY

Painful Suffering from Neuropathy 75% Relieved within Days:
https://www.youtube.com/watch?v=WBjchfwi1jA

Blast with This, Or, Bathe
with That

So what I had been doing for most of my life, like most people in the developed world, was eating a typical Western diet that was hurting my body relentlessly at every meal with fat, cholesterol, processed foods, and toxins which were creating inflammation, chronic pain and oxidative stress not to mention other direct damage.

Dr. Caldwell Esselstyn of the Cleveland Clinic says that with each meal of the typical Western diet people are blasting their systems with foods that cause injury, but that because the body is very good at fixing itself, it can recover, he estimates 90%, but then the next snack or meal comes along and causes another injury, and then the body recovers 90% again. But over time these constant injurious blasts take their toll.

Dr. Esselstyn explains:
https://www.youtube.com/watch?v=o84UcG1p_MA

Just like someone who does a repetitive motion for many years may wear out some of their joints, we wear out our insides prematurely.

Now I try to bathe my insides with really good things that help my body restore itself and fight inflammation, premature aging, cardiovascular damage, cancer, and tumor growth.

As I've mentioned, about every 100 days our cells regenerate, so the question I ask myself is, "Do I want to feed or fight my body and cells as they try to do their job?"

It is never too late to do the right thing! Dr. Esselstyn at the Cleveland Clinic has proven with his scientifically valid studies, our bodies are amazing enough to use the right substances to repair previous damage.

Antioxidant Rich Foods with Every Meal
https://www.youtube.com/watch?v=onH9lK-Mi5mc&list=PL5TLzNi5fYd_yyFvli1diAunJvcJ7x3YX&index=6

Antioxidant Power of Plant Foods:
https://www.youtube.com/watch?v=mg7dyj7p2W-M&list=PL5TLzNi5fYd_yyFvli1diAunJvcJ7x3YX&index=10

Food Antioxidants and Cancer
https://www.youtube.com/watch?v=gvodHKXH0X-U&list=PL5TLzNi5fYd_yyFvli1diAunJvcJ7x3YX&index=5

Minimum Recommended Daily Allowance of Antioxidants
https://www.youtube.com/watch?v=yVjTKBw7_To&list=PL5TLzNi5fYd_yyFvli1diAunJvcJ7x3YX&index=7

Antioxidant Content of 300 Foods
https://www.youtube.com/watch?v=ss6bwKdOgXg

Most People Have an Antioxidant Deficiency
https://www.youtube.com/watch?v=qnHQO4L7Ajo

Opportunity to Bathe in Antioxidants Around the Clock
https://www.youtube.com/watch?v=7nz5Kza9Bqg

Only a Few Weeks Away from Results and Feeling Better

The amazing thing is that you could be only a few weeks away from feeling better and being on a path to being so much healthier.

I know this sounds too good to be true, but I have personally experienced it and people who know me and have seen me almost always remark how great I am looking these days. You can get the same results.

How quickly can you reduce your cholesterol on a plant based diet?
https://www.youtube.com/watch?v=ZTnbND_MpRA&t=88s

Getting Started on Your Journey

- Cut out dairy. This is easy for me because there are satisfactory alternatives.
- Cut out eggs. They are hand grenades that were being tossed at me loaded with saturated fat, cholesterol, choline, arachidonic acid and some other bad stuff. Even egg whites have some of the bad stuff. And because of the way they are raised, you risk exposing yourself to disease pathogens such as the following that are shared between poultry and humans:
    - Avian influenza(Bird flu)
    - Campylobacteriosis is an infection by the Campylobacter bacterium, most commonly C. jejuni. It is among the most common bacterial infections of humans, often a foodborne illness. It produces an inflammatory, sometimes bloody, diarrhea or dysentery syndrome, mostly including cramps, fever and pain.
    - E. coli
    - Salmonella
    - West Nile Virus
- Eat at least a cup of legumes a day: beans, peas, len-

tils edamame, can be worked into: tacos, burritos, stir-frys, or noodle dishes like pad thai, easy.

– Cut out fast food. It's a "Diabetes Express Lane."

– Cut out processed foods. They are mostly made with refined ingredients that race into your system wreaking havoc, often times with nasty high fructose corn syrup.

– Chew, Chew, Chew: sorry no juicing, and limit smoothies. Once again these are forms of processing. Cut it out and eat the old-fashioned way: chew.

– Fiber Up!   Crank up the grams per day to what our bodies evolved to process. Try to get to at least 50 grams a day. But make this change gradually to give your system time to adjust.

– Label check: Do not buy or consume anything with high fructose corn syrup or aspartame or sucralose, and go back to sugar, or honey, or molasses on the label if you have to consume a processed packaged product. Don't buy things with added oils if possible, especially coconut oil, palm oil, or any Omega 6 oils.

– Drink at least a half a bottle of water before any meal or snack. Hydration helps so many things.

– Stop drinking soda and juices. Try eating a cup of grapes or an orange or other whole fruit and drink a bottle of water when you are thirsty and need a boost! It makes you feel so much better!!

– Fight cancer with everything you consume. https://www.youtube.com/watch?v=0VX_oZBMSd4

So I Know the Thought of Switching from Familiar Routines and Habits and Going Plant Based is Intimidating for Most to Consider

But I have been where you are. But I did it.

And I want to help you.

Don't think too much about it, don't let it overwhelm you. Just start with some simple steps and ease into it. Baby steps, easy peasy. You really should increase your fiber intake gradually instead of all at once anyway.

Hopefully you have read this far into the book you are ready to make some steps towards better nutrition to give your cells what they want.

It's a process, like most things in life, but it has been worth it for me. One of our cycling & stair climbing friends introduced us to a great saying:
"So how do you get stronger tomorrow???" "You start

today!!!"

In general, the process can be thought of as: Replacing those old habitual piles of food with new and improved piles of food that will take you towards these objectives:

- Foods not processed so they don't "race" into your system.
- Not carrying the baggage of things your body wasn't designed for.
- Help rebuild your gut Microbiome by feeding the good colonies and starving out the bad colonies.
- Bathe your insides with antioxidants.
- Feed your cells with the wide spectrum of nutrients that your body was designed to function with and use to regenerate.
- Wide spectrum of whole complete foods that the amazing body knows how to use, rather than trying to outsmart it by focusing on any particular element of nutrition.

Today is the day you start your journey, here are some simple steps:

- Pour any liquid dairy products that are in your home down the drain.

- Throw out any dairy based yogurt, sour cream, cottage cheese, ice cream.

- Replace the liquid and soft dairy items with cashew, almond, soy, rice or whatever non-dairy products you can readily find.

- Keep your hard cheeses for now, this is a transition.

- Buy some steel cut oats and prepare them for breakfast tomorrow.

- Buy some blueberries, I like the frozen organic ones at Costco or Sam's.

- Big bags of walnuts and almonds from Costco or Sam's are a good deal.

- Buy some bananas and dry roasted nuts to have available for snacks.

- Throw away any processed meats, they are known carcinogens.

- Locate spices for tomorrow's oatmeal: turmeric, black pepper, cinnamon, cloves, ginger, nutmeg or pumpkin pie spice.

- Find something to sweeten your oatmeal tomorrow if preferred: raisins, chopped apples, peaches, nectarines, raisins, honey, real maple syrup, brown sugar if you must, whatever makes you happy!

- Steel cut oats are better than rolled oats and there are two basic reasons: 1) they are lower on the glycemic scale as rolled oats are more processed meaning they go into your system faster, and 2) bits of the steel cut oats are more likely to make it to your lower intestine so that they will feed the good bacteria in your gut to make beneficial things and hopefully crowd out the bad bacteria that used to feed on meat and other animal products that made the harmful TMAO and hydrogen sulfide gas.

Tomorrow Morning and Every Morning Going Forward if Possible:

- Use the non-dairy milk in your coffee if that is how you take it, and for any other purpose where you used to consume dairy milk.

- Make a big bowl of steel cut oats and blueberries, enough to have half for breakfast and the other half for a snack later in the day. Sprinkle spices on it.

- Make the bowl of oats and blueberries as delicious as you can. I add cinnamon, nutmeg, cloves, banana, honey or real maple syrup or even brown sugar, or I use raisins for sweetness, or chop up an apple, or whatever fruit is super fresh at the time, like peaches or nectarines, throw in some walnuts or pecans, etc. Just make the bowl so good you look forward to having half later as a snack.

Sometime During the First Week:

- Look at the ingredients on the items in your fridge and pantry to find any items with "high fructose corn syrup" or "palm oil" or "coconut oil" or any kind of "trans fats," and throw them out, they are putting unnatural garbage into you.

- Replace with ketchup, relish or other products that have sugar, honey, or molasses or something natural on the label instead of HFCS (high fructose corn syrup).

- Replace with peanut butter that has two ingredients: peanuts and salt.

- In general, if you need to buy packaged and processed foods then buy products that have as few ingredients on the labels as possible, and have some fiber, and are low in fat and salt, with no dairy or eggs.

- Pick up some hummus and something crunchy to dip into it for snacks. Avoid fried crunchy things and look for low fat. I like the Organic Triscuits® from Costco for when I need some crunch. They have very few ingredients.

- Start drinking a bit more water if you can because you are getting more fiber and without water it can cause discomfort. With water it should be very helpful.

- If you need a snack, a banana or any piece of whole fruit, or a bunch of grapes along with a small half handful of nuts should be your snack, with some water or tea.

- Cold steep some Green or Hibiscus Tea and have it available to drink in the fridge when you are thirsty. I like Raspberry Zinger Tea which includes hibiscus.

Second Week:

-   Stop eating eggs by themselves. If you have to make a cake or something, go ahead and use eggs, but try to limit your intake.

-   Make lunches meat free meals. And to make it easy so it won't take a lot of your time. Read the next three bullet points for suggestions on how to get this food quickly without any prep time.

-   I suggest going to Chipotle for lunch and order a vegetarian burrito bowl. I have them make a bed of lettuce, a very small amount of rice, add beans, (I like both the black and the brown beans), Pico de Gallo, sautéed onions and peppers, corn, and guacamole, and more lettuce if there is room. Chipotle is fast and inexpensive and in my experience a meal like this will not bring you down with any after lunch sluggishness. Depending on how big of a person you are you might get a snack or part of a second meal out of the bowl.

-   The next day have a veggie stir fry at an Asian restaurant. You can just go veggie or you can start to try different variations with add ins like tofu or seitan or tempeh. Ask for no egg to be cooked into the dishes like some places do. Skip the fried egg rolls even if they are vegetarian and try to limit the white rice. Fresh spring rolls with no meat are good and brown rice is better if they have it.

- The following day go to a grocery store with a good quality salad bar and make yourself a G.B.O.M.B. salad to include: Greens, Beans, Onions, Mushrooms, and Berries. Seeds and Beets would be great too.

- Eat this way for lunch for a week and then let your imagination and taste buds think of other variations on these themes.

- Start trying to limit your oil intake, even of "healthy" oils. Try not to eat any deep fried foods.

Third Week:
- Keep doing the breakfast thing, but use your imagination if necessary to vary it and keep it interesting with different fruits, spices etc. Buy some vegan chocolate chips if you have to in order to keep the steel cut oats flowing into your body.

- Buy some sprouted grain bread and enjoy it with peanut butter and jam all melted on toast if you need something different for breakfast.

- Keep doing the lunch thing rotating veggie burritos, stir-frys, GBOMB salads, and add veggie burgers into the mix to keep things interesting.

- Eliminate meat from dinner every other day. Use Yelp! Or another search engine to find restaurants that serve veggie and or vegan dishes and go out and taste new foods. It will be fun exploring a whole new world.

- Any day you do still eat meat or animal products of any kind you should eat at least two pieces of fruit, have at least a side salad, and preferably have a serving of something really healthy like cabbage, sauerkraut, broccoli, Brussel sprouts, or cauliflower alongside the meat to "push" it through your gut.

- Check out the Lightlife® and Tofurkey® substitute meat products at the local store and see if any of them look interesting to you. I use them sometimes to make a "comfort food" snack or meal that will make me feel satisfied. Hot dogs, burgers, tacos, "ham" sandwich, burritos, sloppy joes, sausage, etc.

- I buy really good condiments and buns or tortillas and load them down with toppings etc. to make them really good. To be honest, the underlying "meat" being different from the old days is really not very noticeable.

Third Weekend:
- Schedule 2 to 3 hours where you can cook 2 or 3 easy dishes selected from the list of YouTube video recipes that I have listed below. Put what you make and don't eat immediately into storage containers of some type for the refrigerator. These will be for use during week 4.

- Buy or make some hummus for spreading and dipping.

- Prep vegetables and buy oil free non fried chips or crackers for dipping.

- Stock up on canned beans of all types you like, avocados, tortillas, lettuce, tomato, onion, salsa, Pico de Gallo, cilantro if you like it.

- Buy frozen veggie burgers to have on hand, buy some good buns with no egg and with fiber; sprouted grain baked goods are the best.

- Sprouted grain English muffins are a good addition.

- Buy some good condiments and hot sauces etc. of whatever will make your taste buds happy, and vegan mayo if you like mayo.

- Buy some vegan butter and cheese to try it out. I cut it out mostly later when I went further to oil free.

- Buy granola, nuts, seeds like pumpkin, all for snacking whenever.

Fourth Week:
- No more animal products going forward. Hopefully the additional fiber that has been introduced into your diet for the first few weeks is working to transition your digestive tract.

- This is when your body should really start to transition and feel better.

- Keep going with the steel cut oats and berries if possible, if not for breakfast then for a snack. Oats do so many good things.

- One meal during the day should center around "greens", like a big yummy GBOMB salad or some derivative.

- Don't hesitate to snack as much as is necessary to get yourself through each day, snack with whole foods, nuts, fruits, veggies or Triscuits® and hummus.

- Peanut butter and jam will get you through a meal or snack.

- Keep some frozen veggie burgers on hand for meals or snacks.

- Guacamole is a food group.

- Tortillas with black beans, salsa, guacamole, and anything else is a quick easy satisfying meal or snack.

- I ate constantly during this time to keep myself satisfied but yet I still lost weight. On plant based nutrition you need to make sure you are getting sufficient calories anyway or there is a chance you won't feel good and you will give up or fail, so eat, eat, eat!

- If you are eating a wide spectrum of plant based foods, preferably whole foods, and you are getting sufficient calories, you should be getting everything your body needs.

- The exception is B-12, Buy some vitamin B-12 and take it daily.

Fifth thru Seventh Weeks:
- Keep it going, animal products free if at all possible, to try to get the bad stuff out of your system

- I batch cook every five days or so to keep a supply of good food in containers in the fridge for grab and go convenience.

- I like bananas so there are always some around for quick snacks.

- If you have an off day, it is ok, but don't consider it a failure or a setback. It happens, especially in the early days. Just get back to it at the next meal or snack, don't give up, it will be worth it.

- So by now you will hopefully be fully plant based for at least three weeks. At three weeks I had lost about seven pounds and was feeling better. I was still a bit gassy as my gut was transitioning and still dealing with the extra fiber. That's normal. Just keep on your journey.

– Keep looking for more restaurants that support plant based eating and keep trying the recipes on the videos. Most of them I have suggested do not require very much time, the people in the videos are fun, and it is really enjoyable to know what is going into your food and taking control of your health.

For recipes, see the end of the book. Now in case you need more evidence, following are some additional reasons why Veganism makes so much sense as a dietary choice, and more encouragement for your journey:

When Your Body Needs to Send in the Marines

Make sure your immune system's white blood cell fighters are ready and up to the tasks at hand.

There are two platoons of white blood cells: B and T. But these important cells weaken with age, and malfunction. B cells lose their vigor in attacking bacteria, viruses, and cancer cells, and the T cells lose their vigor in attacking cells foreign to the body, such as cancer cells and transplant cells.

Even worse is when B and T cells malfunction, they attack normal healthy body cells.

Damage to the bone marrow can reduce their production. Smoking tobacco is the most common way to damage bone marrow over the long term.

There are things I consume to boost these cells and keep them ready for action: Blueberries, raspberries, blackberries, or one of my favorites: Seaweed Salad.

Boosting Natural Killer Cells with Nutrition:

https://www.youtube.com/watch?v=FGtS_h_xTuc&t=168s

Which Berries are the Best? :
https://www.youtube.com/watch?v=Xp_lb_Pe7gE

Try to prevent damage to your Bone Marrow.
Bone marrow is the spongy tissue inside bones that produces blood cells. Bone marrow produces red blood cells, platelets, and white blood cells. Lymphocytes are produced in the marrow, and play an important part in the body's immune system.
https://nutritionfacts.org/topics/blood-cancer/

Things I am Mindful of:

- The beef industry has a bigger marketing budget than the broccoli industry.

- "White" meat is still full of saturated fat and cholesterol and has bio-accumulated toxins even if it is free range or organic or just landed from Mars.

- Most animals raised for consumption were raised in their own filth.

- Toxins: First limit what gets into or onto your body and then try to facilitate elimination via discharge. Fiber is one of the most important things in discharging toxins!

Dividend Reinvestment Plan:

Once I realized how inexpensive it is to enjoy plant based nutrition, I started to reinvest my savings by selecting foods labeled as organic and without high fructose corn syrup, artificial sweeteners, palm oil, coconut oil or anything that really looks unnatural.

Are Organic Foods Healthier?
https://www.youtube.com/watch?v=lkgs3xIN1HM

Are Organic Foods Safer?
https://www.youtube.com/watch?v=6Icpg2RWgZE

Which Foods Contain the Most Pesticides?
https://www.youtube.com/watch?v=IUSfV2p9frI

Is Organic Meat Less Carcinogenic?
https://www.youtube.com/watch?v=aSHv5vDi3Is

What about Kosher and Organic Chicken?
https://www.youtube.com/watch?v=RyP5Cnc-vxk

Beggar on the Box

There was once a beggar sitting at the front of a building on a little wooden box. For years he sat in the same spot, asking people who passed by for small coins. Then one day someone asked him what was in the box he was sitting on each day.

The beggar had no idea, but curious himself, he looked, and found the box was full of gold! All the years he had been asking for handouts, he actually had all the resources he could ever need.

We are just like that beggar. We have been looking for quick solutions to be given to us too. We want better health and we want it to be easy. But all the while we are all sitting on a box full of gold in our own bodies, which will take good care of us, if we just feed it well.

We don't need to wait to get sick and for the medical industry to discover or invent solutions, because the gold is within our reach.

The power to steer onto a better path is with us.

The challenge and intention of this book is to get you and all the people I care about to realize something very powerful is within your own reach.

Is Medicine Going to Fix You?

Some people think that if they have an incurable disease that they could be frozen in suspended animation until science comes up with a cure.

Most of the drug companies and medical researchers are not looking for cures they are looking for things to sell. They are looking to isolate molecules that they can then package and sell as therapies.

I think you will have trouble finding any medicine that is a path to a cure.

If you start to take a medicine there is a very good chance you are going to take it for the rest of your life which is fully in step with the goals of the big corporations who need to make their quarterly numbers and enhance shareholder value. That is what corporations do.

There are a handful of doctors out there like Esselstyn of the Cleveland Clinic who have decades of evidence of arresting and reversing disease.

Basically this is giving your body the plant based nutrients that it had evolved to use to take care of itself as the body is a very powerful healer if it is only given the right nutrients. The cells then regenerate every 100 days so you are 3 months away from feeling better and looking better if you just give your body the chance.

My 85 year old mother who takes 12 to 15 pills a day and can barely make it to the bathroom with a walker asked me why I was doing this. My answer was that I cannot afford to eat the way I used to, and it isn't that I don't have the money, but it is that I don't have the time to end up like she has sick and on multiple medications.

I used to worry about running out of money when I got old. But now I only worry about running out of time to do things, because I am healthy.

I can't afford to eat animal products because they're too expensive, because they will cost me my good health.

It isn't just how long I'm going to live, it's also how well I'm going to live. I am going to try to be healthy as long as I can and not be the grandparent or great grandparent that somebody has to push around in a wheelchair or help to and from the car.

I want to be able to walk up to my seat when I see my granddaughter graduate from high school and college and then who knows maybe even when I see her children graduate from high school or college. I want to still be able to walk and to not be in pain. Those are the goals I'm trying to reach.

I start my day with a bowl of energy not a plate of fat and cholesterol.
A plate of fat and cholesterol like bacon-and-eggs and toast and butter will most likely make me feel like I want to go back to bed because it will sap my energy.

One of my rules of thumb now is if I eat something that makes me feel like I want to go lay down then I probably ate the wrong thing—food should be energizing.

Treating the consequences versus the causes is what most people do by relying on medicine.

Eat for energy and nutrients, not for a quick satisfying mouthfeel of fat and salt.

I find my bowl of steel cut oats and blueberries, bananas and apples to be extremely satisfying. It makes me feel good and really sets me for the morning with a positive spin on things.

Even if someone is not going to stop eating animal products they get a lot of benefits from increasing fruit and vegetable consumption, especially if they can get fiber per day up to 50 grams.

Insurance companies use population data and the science of statistics to improve their profits, so people should not ignore the data and the science to improve their health.....
Health is Wealth.

And let's say there is a type of brakes that are suspected for not working properly and may be causing accidents.

So if a study was done to show they were okay and it was funded by the brake manufacturer or the manufacturer's group I would think no one would even think twice about the fact that it should be questioned as to whether it was valid or not.

Yet there are studies out there on nutrition funded by the egg board and the dairy industry and the beef industry and the pork industry and the chicken industry that get into popular periodicals like women's health and on the 6 o'clock news and they give people just enough rational-ization power to continue to consume things that indepen-dent studies show are not beneficial for our health.

Penny Stocks

Most people dream of investing in a stock like McDonalds or Google when it was a "penny stock" and then riding it up to great wealth.

Come over here and let me whisper an insider tip to you.

What if I told you I know a company that is coming out with a prescription that has through valid scientific clinical trials been shown to halt and reverse heart disease, cancer, intestinal diseases, diabetes and a number of other chronic conditions?

And it only costs pennies to invest in this company ... you would want to know the ticker symbol so you could place an order immediately.

This is that penny stock. The ticker symbol is PBN—Plant Based Nutrition.

Health is wealth. I have a huge incentive to increase my own profits. That is how our capitalistic society functions in that each person works to increase their income and lower their risks and costs.

My Story

I have been where most people are now. I ate just like everyone else, probably worse. I didn't go out of my way to eat fruits and veggies. I hated oatmeal.

Let me run through a typical day of my eating choices back then.

Breakfast.....
- Bacon and waffles
- Sausage and butter sandwiches
- Cheese omelet with hash browns
- Croissants, plain, ham and cheese, chocolate
- Fried eggs with bacon or sausage and toast
- Cereal with white sugar and milk
- Cereal with lots of brown sugar and milk

Mid morning snack:
- Doughnuts
- Bagel and cream cheese
- Leftover pizza
- Breakfast sandwich, hash browns and OJ at drive thru
- Breakfast sandwich with ham usually and OJ at

drive thru

Lunch:
- Burgers and fries and soda
- Hot dogs, fries and soda
- Pizza slices and soda
- Italian beef and fries and soda
- Gyros and fries and soda
- You get the picture

Afternoon snack:
- Any or all of the above

Dinner:
- Steak, potatoes, salad, soup, soda
- Fried chicken, potatoes, cole slaw, soda
- Pizza with sausage or pepperoni or both

Evening Snack:
- Any or all of the above

Midnight Snack:
- Any or all of the above

This was every day, not kidding, every day, massive ingestion of the foods most people eat.

So by the time I was 40 years old I was 272 pounds. While I was never out of breath, I would sweat for a while even after a moderate walk through an airport.

I had to find a potty to sit on at least 6 times a day, and with hemorrhoids, it wasn't pleasant. I'll spare you the details.

I had gout attacks, painful, crazy painful gout attacks. Life kind of sucked.

The doctor wanted me to take multiple medications for my health issues.

I had gone from a young strong man unloading railcars and trucks at age 17 to a fragile adult in chronic pain at age 40 who was about to start taking pills for the rest of his life. Not exactly good times.

So I decided I didn't want to take pills every day for the rest of my life so I started looking for other things to try. That journey led me here. I hope it helps you too, to find a level of health and vitality uncommon to most Americans.

Handling Holidays

There are happy associations with food that we as a culture have evolved to think are important. And I am not saying they are not. There are comfort foods, family celebrations and memories that center around pressure to make some really bad food choices.

And maybe once in a while these foods are ok to celebrate or to remember and enjoy life.

But it is my experience, and what actual science shows, is that these kinds of foods mess with our metabolic processes and biochemistry because these are not things our body is engineered to process.

Improved Performance and Shortened Recovery Time

Bodybuilding:
https://www.vice.com/en_us/article/8qgzvg/how-to-get-ripped-on-a-vegan-diet

Six Reasons for Athletes:
https://www.pcrm.org/news/blog/six-reasons-athletes-are-running-toward-vegan-diet

Tom Brady:
https://www.peta.org/living/food/tom-brady-plant-based-meals/

Gronk Follows Brady:
https://www.livekindly.com/patriots-rob-gronkowski-tom-brady-vegan-meals/

Yale Test 1907 :
https://nutritionfacts.org/video/the-first-studies-on-vegetarian-athletes/

Improving Performance and Recovery:

https://www.youtube.com/watch?v=bfERQJLvo6A

Some Wisdom I Have Come Across in My Observations:

What I've learned is that I am really the only one who has the ability to be responsible for my own health. I chose not to wait until society catches up with the information and data about the dangers of eating the typical Western diet.

I know that I will die someday, I just do not want it to be my own fault.

Doctors for the most part don't seem to know any more about nutrition than the general public. I watched many doctors, their spouses and families eat at my restaurant for many years, so I have decided to not wait until my doctor "kicks the habit": https://youtu.be/6D6vbXH-tAc

I feel so good these days I really believe I have created and am living in my own personal Blue Zone: https://www.youtube.com/watch?v=zmYygsxoR9o

Why Am I So Passionate About This?

I am passionate about healthy nutrition because I am passionate about my family. I have 3 children (and their beloved wonderful partners, and a grandchild and one more on the way). I want them to have this information to consider, at an age that I wish I had had it.

Because I feel way better at 60 than I did at 40, I want to share how I got here. I feel so light and flexible and full of energy. That first trip down the stairs in the morning when I used to feel some stiffness in my knees and feet is totally gone. I feel like a youngster again.

People keep telling me how good I am looking these days (must have looked really bad before), and how good the results from my blood tests have been.

My little buddy Mandy was doing so great for the last couple of years of her life and was pretty darn healthy up until 16 and a half years of age. It seemed to be from feeding her plant based foods that had been recommended by the Bichon rescue lady. That wasn't proof of course, but it got me to thinking about the subject and questioning things.

I'm passionate about this because 60 for my dad and 67 for Granny was too young to die. Both events took away from my life, and I wish I had found this information and framework of thought 20 years ago when I had health issues and started to look for solutions.

And I want to share this to help people. I've been a selfish person most of my life and it is time I really tried to help people, especially my children and Aubrey and Phil Jr.

I feel by now my gut microbiome has changed which, according to the science, should be changing the chemicals that are floating around my body and brain.

My evidence of this is twofold: 1) I don't seem to be generating hydrogen sulfide gas as my intestinal gas and bowel movements no longer have that "rotten egg" smell associated with hydrogen sulfide (which is a poison gas by the way), and 2) I seem calmer and less irritable which is consistent with what the science says about TMAO floating around the brain.

Closing Message

"Twenty years from now you will be more disappointed by the things you didn't do than by the ones you did do. So throw off the bowlines. Sail away from the safe harbor." - **Mark Twain**

Also by Mark Twain: "Never regret anything that makes you smile."

Looking in the mirror at my less fat self, and waking up with energy, and feeling light on my feet, and having great bathroom visits, and having great numbers when I get blood tests, and knowing I am playing my hand on the right side of the odds, and knowing I am giving myself a fighting chance to make it to the high school graduations of my grandchildren … all these things make me smile!!

https://www.youtube.com/watch?v=036tJ3uCnPg

Health is truly wealth, and this is a frugal path to the best kind of wealth, which is feeling as good as you can for as many days of life as you can.

I Did Not Want to Change

Someone told a friend of mine, who had destructive behavior patterns, "When you hurt enough, you'll stop." This was true for me too. I didn't want to change. But I didn't want to hurt or be sick anymore.

I am a glutton. I spent most of my life searching for the next best things to indulge in so:

- I wish I could fly and that gravity wasn't true.
- I wish drinking too much didn't cause hangovers or eventually liver problems.
- I wish I could eat big ole juicy Italian beef sandwiches and fries every day for lunch.
- I wish I could eat sausage pizza and potato chips and dip for dinner every night.
- I wish smoking, which I used to do, did not cause me to ingest and absorb toxins like Benzene.

But I got tired of jumping from one new health fad to the next and decided to dig and dig until I found real science. I am learning more every day because I am somewhat obsessed with this knowledge, but I think I have really found where the real science is that most people don't see or don't want to acknowledge.

I wish I could eat and drink whatever I wanted and still feel good and be healthy. But I got sick in a several ways and hated it.

Now I just want to do what I can to try and help people make informed decisions and to get past the clutter of the seemingly conflicting information.

If after reviewing the facts, you want to take your chances with whatever food you want to eat, or with modern medicine being able to take care of possible future issues, then that is fine. But I challenge you to join me on this journey to shoot for the best outcomes.

Two of the richest guys I know, financially, are also the sickest, and they are not that old. It is so obviously from the rich foods they consume, because I have personally seen how they eat. Don't let this happen to you. Don't let your life's blessings become a curse to your health.

I am a poor guy who eats a lot of bean burritos (thankfully I love bean burritos) and feels light on my feet and has good blood test numbers.

I am not a trained nutritional, health, or medical professional of any kind. But a self-studying, self-digging, self-training nutritional biochemistry science geek.

All the Best! Good Luck! (But don't count on just luck, play the odds)

Recipes, as promised:

W hen I started, during my transition, and even to this day, I use videos from YouTube to learn how to make fast and easy plant based foods. They are also usually great sources of information and encouragement.

Here are some of the recipes I have used and enjoyed:

Easy and Fast Pad Thai in 5 Minutes:
https://www.youtube.com/watch?v=g-3po-BTKig

5 Minute Indian Dahl:
https://www.youtube.com/watch?v=Jpq6puQleJ0

Simple Thai Green Curry from Scratch:
https://www.youtube.com/watch?v=7qgX0fVCZ9k

Thai Red Curry
https://www.youtube.com/watch?v=QO1EWD205cY

Best Damn Easy Chili:
https://www.youtube.com/watch?v=9elMtWQ-Ly0

Easy Oats and Fruit Bowl Breakfast Demo:
https://www.youtube.com/watch?v=RcJ9pXctoB0

Three Easy Breakfast Ideas:
https://www.youtube.com/watch?v=6W9cECRPxYU

Breakfast Burrito
https://www.youtube.com/watch?v=6DO3M9ajCOE

Vegan Mac and Cheese:
https://www.youtube.com/watch?v=NxjybJoSms8

Cheesy Cauliflower Broccoli Soup
https://www.youtube.com/watch?v=hXuA7qkC-Ss

West African Peanut Lentil Soup
https://www.youtube.com/watch?v=HUTYDMGSd-c

5 Minute Chickpea Curry
https://www.youtube.com/watch?v=aP6eXpwIths

Mushroom Stroganoff Linguini
https://www.youtube.com/watch?v=kftI9DE5H3o

Peanut Butter Stew
https://www.youtube.com/watch?v=dmGneN9FPjU

South African Chakalaka
https://www.youtube.com/watch?v=Sv1luldeNz4

Chocolate Banana Dessert
https://www.youtube.com/watch?v=NNPEnEy-viQ

Lasagna
https://www.youtube.com/watch?v=M6eVRYX2h1E

Thai Slaw
https://www.youtube.com/watch?v=DHFiZrSYXMM

Zucchini Bread
https://www.youtube.com/watch?v=bCtqu-dUvwc

Oat Waffles
https://www.youtube.com/watch?v=6CSMorgl8SU

Banana Bread
https://www.youtube.com/watch?v=egtDQs_lLJc

Hummus
https://www.youtube.com/watch?v=MQ11Cu4inZI

Easy Caesar Salad Dressing
https://www.youtube.com/watch?v=-6YO3JXRra0

5 Minute Pesto Pasta
https://www.youtube.com/watch?v=5jJNo1CHdQE

5 Minute Meatball Sub Sandwiches
https://www.youtube.com/watch?v=C_kHMJZ9oWI

5 Minute Falafel
https://www.youtube.com/watch?v=FsfncCvu274

Nutritarian Meal Prep for the Week
https://www.youtube.com/watch?v=uYDBxi8vDAU

Roasted Vegetable Pasta
https://www.youtube.com/watch?v=ICdvMev2Poo

5 Minute Buddha Bowl
https://www.youtube.com/watch?v=DqpSoGzwCBo

5 Minute Burgers
https://www.youtube.com/watch?v=r6ZIiiBilOc

Ultimate Veggie Burgers
https://www.youtube.com/watch?v=fsNk68nRS6w

Vegan Burrito in 5 Minutes
https://www.youtube.com/watch?v=0lDjSFhNsE8

Perfect Hummus 3 Ways
https://www.youtube.com/watch?v=ep5CdVvKIo8

Vegan Cream Cheese for Bagels
https://www.youtube.com/watch?v=QJ6oRGs3mZk

Easy Cashew Mayonnaise
https://www.youtube.com/watch?v=y7HLFVEsx9k

Vegan Ice Cream
https://www.youtube.com/watch?v=GskNlVKw9sc

Helpful information, thoughts and tips:

Where can I go out to eat and have plant based nutritional food?
https://www.peta.org/living/food/chain-restaurants/

Taco Bell?
If it was something you consumed during your formative years, it may be one of your "comfort foods".

I get an occasional taste for it myself, usually if I am traveling home from my favorite brewery and I get the munchies ... there is one right on the way.

Taco Bell bean burritos are supposedly vegan, which means their beans do not have lard in them like some restaurants. At many locations you can choose black beans instead of the standard refried beans. Of course you need to leave off the cheese and sour cream.

I find a couple of their black bean burritos with no cheese and no sour cream and the sauce of my choice, lots of it, takes care of my Taco Bell fix and satisfies my munchies and gets me home "safely" past the gauntlet of fast food drive thrus after I have had a few beverages and am susceptible to making bad food choices.

The other thing I do is pre-buy a bottle of Taco Bell Sauce at the grocery store and have it in the fridge at home ready to put on a black bean and hummus and onions and peppers and lettuce and tomato and rice and or or or whatever you like on your favorite tortilla (one with fiber is better than not as every gram helps over the course of a day) to make a very satisfying snack or meal.

Crazy Girl:
https://www.youtube.com/watch?v=dNeaf2m_vyA

Chipotle
At Chipotle I can get a very good and satisfying burrito or burrito bowl with brown and or black beans and brown or white rice and corn and tomatoes and guacamole and sautéed onions and peppers and some lettuce and put some of that yummy tabasco, green, regular and or chipotle and I have had a quick, handy, very satisfying meal for about seven bucks on the go just about anywhere. I don't miss the cheese or sour cream; the guac adds all the creaminess I need.

Silly Girl:
https://www.youtube.com/watch?v=6DSnNx5CgEY

Thai

Thai curries are really easy to make, and I now make them all the time, but I love to cook.

Thai restaurants are everywhere and they offer such flavorful and satisfying dishes and they always seem very understanding and helpful when making sure what they serve you has no animal products in it.

Panang curry with just vegetables (or add Tofu, or every once in a while they have seitan) is so satisfying and creamy and with a side of steamed broccoli to dip into it is going to make your body and mind very happy.

Pad Thai usually has egg stirred and fried into it so be careful to ask that they leave it out unless you are just going to have an off day … which I get once in a while … Just don't be surprised if you feel funny after eating high fat eggs or meat or cheese after you have been off them for a while … or if your nose breaks out a couple of days later.

Snacking Constantly

Snack, snack, snack, it's okay to snack! In what I am doing I do not count calories I just eat when I'm hungry. When I think I am hungry I first drink a bottle of water and often that takes care of some of the hunger. If you're still hungry—eat!

Snack Ideas:
https://www.youtube.com/watch?v=VNPWeLprHUk

Drinks

Drinking enough water is essential for physiological processes such a circulation metabolism temperature regulation and waste removal.

Even mild dehydration can cause issues such as headaches, irritability, poor physical performance, and reduction in cognitive function.

How much water should we drink?:
https://www.youtube.com/watch?v=qrzSLIBOauM

Alkaline Water:
https://www.youtube.com/watch?v=wpYO_3nTsNo

Bottled Water versus Tap:
https://www.youtube.com/watch?v=k--vSmBZKPo

Lead in Our Drinking Water:
https://www.youtube.com/watch?v=bZnvbriXGrI

Supplements Versus the Real Thing (Fruits, Veggies, Etc)

Supplements Review:
https://nutritionfacts.org/topics/supplements/

Should We Take a Multivitamin?:
https://www.youtube.com/watch?v=5fgVDT0qw88

Throw Away Your Supplements:
https://www.youtube.com/watch?v=3NlKGlMoUow&pb-jreload=10

Frugality

Anyone who knows me, knows I am quite frugal. Why spend the money on expensive animal products loaded with cholesterol only to then have to spend money on drugs to manage the cholesterol???

Bigger Bang for your Bucks:
https://www.youtube.com/watch?v=QOn1hVZUDvo

So You Think You Are Fit?
https://www.youtube.com/watch?v=L3oZ3lPvGTE

I Now Get to Enjoy the Comfort Foods I Grew Up with:

For a number of years I stopped eating many of the "comfort foods" that I grew up eating like hamburgers, hot dogs, tacos, chili, chili dogs, breakfast sausage, Italian sausage, etc.

Mac n Cheese:
https://www.youtube.com/watch?v=wPD-IFecwbU

I eat hot dogs, burgers, tacos, chili, etc. because there are ways to make all these things in delicious ways that do not include ground up dead animals.

Now that I realize there are plant based foods that can be made to have similar textures and flavors, seasoned with the same seasonings (plant based) that are used to season the beef, pork and chicken I used to eat. And the resulting foods are lower in fat and have no cholesterol.

I get to eat hot dogs, chili dogs, Italian sausage with roasted peppers on French rolls, breakfast sausage, all of which I had stopped eating several years ago.

Are these the healthiest forms of plant based foods? Not really, but they are better than the animal based versions and I am happy by satisfying my desire for the comfort foods I grew up with.

Even though I promised I would not try to tell anyone what to do … My dream is to get my loved ones and friends, and anybody who will listen to:

Try It! Experience It!   There are no harmful side effects, only the chance to feel better, look better, and to give yourself the best chance to live a long and pain free life.

The stiffness in my feet, knees and legs in general is gone, my acne has cleared up, I have lost weight, and I have not thought about taking Ibuprofen for 24 months.

Yet I know people my age or even younger who can barely walk, and it breaks my heart.

Even if you can give it a try for a few weeks to see how you feel, this is a path that can make you healthier.

The path of medicine that most people are on never seems to make them better. They will take the medicine forever, and more of it. I am 62 and take no medicine.

You don't even have to quit your medicines to try it, but I have heard stories of diabetics who have chosen this path that had to be quickly taken off their medications because their numbers improved so rapidly … like in a few weeks. So be careful, this can have dramatic results in as quickly as a few weeks.

If You Do Nothing Else: Simply Add Some Fruits, Vegetables and Flax

If you do absolutely nothing else based upon this book, please consider eating at least five servings of fruits and veggies a day to up your fiber to a better range and to get what seems to be the optimal level of vitamin C into your bloodstream which has significant anti-cancer effects.

Rather than taking a vitamin C supplement the absorption into your body is better if you actually eat the foods containing the vitamin C.

This seems to work with a lot of things. Isolated supplements don't seem to get absorbed into the body as well as when you eat the whole food. You are what you absorb!
https://www.health.harvard.edu/staying-healthy/should-you-get-your-nutrients-from-food-or-from-supplements
https://nutritionfacts.org/topics/supplements/

Work a spoonful or two of ground flaxseed into your food somewhere each day. Omega-3 fatty acids are so beneficial and necessary and flaxseed is a great source.

Eight or nine servings of fruits and vegetables a day, and a serving of a whole grain like steel cut oatmeal, and at least one serving of a legume like black beans, and a tablespoon of ground flaxseed together are getting almost to optimal for supplying all the nutrients and fiber you need!

Reversing Diabetes and Pre Diabetes:
https://www.youtube.com/watch?v=bVmjcIoJZWQ

https://www.youtube.com/watch?v=CbVflDOWCbU

Into My Third Year: Where I am Trying to Improve

I think I've done pretty well. It seems my gut microbiome has transitioned as I am no longer producing smelly gas, and my tummy is flatter, and I don't feel any bloating after I eat.

As I look in the mirror, I see a guy who is no longer puffy with inflammation.

But I am not perfect. I am still a glutton or have some kind of food addiction issues going on: I just love to eat!

So here, based on the science I am continuing to dig for and study, are some things I am trying to do better and more consistently:

- Move from black bean burgers to black beans.(more whole foods)
- Less bread, both solid (bread) and liquid (beer). (less processed)
- Expand variety of food sources.(build up more diverse microbiome)
- Stop eating when I am 80% full.(portion control)

- Eliminate late night snacks.(can disturb peaceful sleep)
- Supplement with plant derived Omega-3 EPA/DHA.(brain health)
- Supplement with both kinds of B-12 just to be safe.
- Exercise more vigorously, not just being active. (work up to a sweat)
- Work to sleep better and longer.(sleep is good!)
- Enjoy more passion and intimacy; love and be loved.
- Finish this gosh darn book I have been messing with for too long!

Please for yourself and your own well being and feeling good every day, consider giving Plant Based Nutrition a three week try!
And I Sincerely believe, from my own experience that you will be amazed!!!